MEDICAL
INTELLIGENCE
UNIT

MALIGNANT MELANOMAS: ADVANCES IN TREATMENT

Stanley P. L. Leong, M.D.

University of California, San Francisco

R.G. LANDES COMPANY
AUSTIN

R.G. LANDES COMPANY
Austin / Georgetown

CRC Press is the exclusive worldwide distributor all Medical Intelligence Unit publications.
CRC Press, 2000 Corporate Blvd., NW, Boca Raton, FL 33431. Phone: 407/994-0555

Submitted: July 1992
Published: September 1992

Managing Editor: Carol Harwell
Production Manager: Terry Nelson
Copy Editor: Constance Kerkaporta

Please address all inquiries to the Publisher:
R.G. Landes Company
909 South Pine Street
Georgetown, TX 78626
or
P.O. Box 4858
Austin, TX 78765
Phone: 512/ 863 7762
FAX: 512/ 863 0081

ISBN 1-879702-26-6
CATALOG LN0226

DEDICATION

This book is dedicated to all the melanoma patients we have treated. They are the true heroes who have inspired us to learn more and more everyday about this challenging disease.

Acknowledgments

We appreciate the secretarial assistance of Lynda Y. Sahlin.

CONTRIBUTORS

Lee S. Albert, M.D.
Massachusetts General Hospital
Boston, Massachusetts

Robert E. Allen, Jr., M.D., F.A.C.S.
Clinical Professor of Surgery
University of California, San Francisco
Attending Surgeon
Mount Zion Medical Center of UCSF
San Francisco, California

Karen K. Fu, M.D.
Professor of Radiation Oncology
University of California
San Francisco Medical Center
San Francisco, California

Evan M. Hersh, M.D.
Professor of Medicine
University of Arizona
Prof. of Immunology/ Microbiology
University of Arizona
Chief, Section of Hematology/Oncology
University of Arizona Cancer Center
Tucson, Arizona

Michele Pruitt Humel, R.R.T., C.C.P.
Perfusionist, Mount Zion Medical Center
University of California, San Francisco
San Francisco, California

John C. Hutchinson, M.D.
Clinical Professor of Medicine/ Surgery
University of California, San Francisco
San Francisco, California

Stanley P.L. Leong, M.D., F.A.C.S.
Associate Professor of Surgery, University
of California, San Francisco
Attending Surgeon, Mount Zion Medical
Center of UCSF
San Francisco, California

Stephen J. Mathes, M.D., F.A.C.S.
Professor of Surgery
Head, Div. of Plastic/Reconstructive Surg.
University of California, San Francisco
San Francisco, California

Richard W. Sagebiel, M.D.
Clinical Prof. of Pathology/Dermatology
University of California, San Francisco
Director, Melanoma Center
Mount Zion Medical Center of UCSF
San Francisco, California

Arthur J. Sober, M.D.
Associate Professor of Dermatology
Harvard Medical School
and Massachusetts General Hospital
Boston, Massachusetts

Patrick S. Swift, M.D.
Assistant Professor of Radiation Oncology
University of California, San Francisco
San Francisco, California

Charles W. Taylor, M.D.
Assistant Professor of Medicine
Section of Hematology/Oncology
University of Arizona
and Arizona Cancer Center
Tucson, Arizona

CONTENTS

PREFACE

The clinical landmarks in predicting the prognosis of malignant melanoma is the adoption of Clark's level and subsequently, Breslow's thickness together with gender of the patient, ulceration and location of the primary. Extensive studies have shown that thin melanoma (<0.9 mm), in general, has a favorable prognosis with a 95% survival over 10 years, and thick melanoma (>1.7 mm) carries a poor prognosis with 45% survival over 10 years. Therefore, microstaging of melanoma is crucial in predicting its clinical outcome and has revolutionized the surgical treatment of melanoma. Dr. Sagebiel's chapter on *Epidemiology and Pathology of Human Malignant Melanoma* sets the tone for the classification and histologic diagnosis of malignant melanoma. Although the incidence of malignant melanoma is rising rapidly, doubling every 10 years, the overall mortality has increased slightly, indicating that most of the melanoma being diagnosed is of the thin level and can be effectively treated by definitive surgical resection. To emphasize the importance of early diagnosis of melanoma so that melanoma in situ or potentially abnormal moles can be removed before they become invasive or high-risk, Drs. Albert and Sober describe in their chapter *Early Diagnostic Approaches for Human Melanoma* the current approaches of early diagnosis of malignant melanoma. When the diagnosis of melanoma is made, it is important for a patient to see a surgeon who specializes in melanoma. I summarize the current approaches in the *Surgical Management of Primary Melanoma*. Based on the thickness of the primary tumor, the re-excision margin can be tailored to individual patients in contrast to the traditional approach of a 5 cm margin for any melanoma. Further, it is the general consensus that no elective lymph node dissection is required for thin melanoma less than 1 mm. For melanoma thicker than 1 mm, the role of elective lymph node dissection is still controversial. When melanoma recurs, such as satellitosis or intransit metastasis limited to the extremities, isolated hyperthermic perfusion may be indicated. Drs. Allen, Hutchinson, Michele Humel and I summarize the therapeutic role of isolated hyperthermic perfusion in the chapter entitled *Isolated Perfusion for Malignant Melanoma*. When melanoma is metastatic in isolated sites, the most effective treatment is to resect if surgically possible. Drs. Allen and Mathes describe the situations and indications for surgical intervention for metastatic melanoma in their chapter entitled *Surgical Treatment of Metastatic Melanoma*. The adjuvant and therapeutic role of radiation therapy for malignant melanoma is discussed by Drs. Swift and Fu in their chapter, *Radiation Treatment of Human Melanoma*. When metastatic melanoma becomes widespread, there is no curable treatment available to date. However, Drs. Taylor and Hersh summarize the currently available chemotherapeutic regimens for the treatment of melanoma in their chapter, *Chemotherapy of Melanoma*. Finally, Drs. Hersh, Taylor and I discuss the impact of biologic modifiers as a new potential modality for the treatment of metastatic melanoma in the chapter *Immunotherapy and Biological Therapy of Malignant Melanoma*.

This monograph emphasizes the need for early diagnosis of melanoma so that it can be eradicated at its earliest stage with an intent of cure. It also demonstrates the significance of microstaging of melanoma upon which surgical treatment depends. Further, it deals with the current and future treatment modalities for local and systemic disease. The chapters are arranged in such a way that the significance of multidisciplinary approaches between the primary physicians, dermatologists, pathologists, surgeons, radiation and medical oncologists is brought into sharp focus. It is the hope of the authors that a melanoma patient is treated in a melanoma center within which all these disciplines are represented. It is in this setting that newer approaches and protocols may be developed so that significant strides may be made to combat this challenging disease.

Stanley P.L. Leong, M.D.
San Francisco, California, 1992

CHAPTER 1

EPIDEMIOLOGY AND PATHOLOGY OF MALIGNANT MELANOMA

Richard W. Sagebiel

There have been remarkable changes in the understanding of malignant melanoma during the past 20 years. The increasing incidence, the relation to precursor lesions, and the ability to recognize different variants of melanoma with their unique biologic behavior has remarkably altered the clinician's ability to deal with this neoplasm .[1,2] The microstage measurements of level of invasion and tumor thickness — together with sex, location and age — are important elements in the evaluation of prognosis. Therefore current therapy recommendations for melanoma should consider these histopathologic parameters.[3-5]

Despite the many changes and advances, however, most can be reduced to the following conclusions: 1) surgery remains the primary mode of therapy for melanoma, 2) the improved survival rate noted in the last 20 years can be attributed largely to excision of thin tumors with better prognosis, and 3) the ability to identify low and high risk groups from clinical and histological features has allowed a more conservative surgical approach to low risk melanoma.

In recent years, the concept of neoplastic transformation as it applies to many human cancers has increased our understanding of the early steps toward malignancy in the melanocytic system.[6,7] Because melanoma is located on the surface of the skin and is generally pigmented, the steps can be recognized and interrupted prior to the development of a neoplasm with any reasonable likelihood of spread. In this chapter the precursor lesions and epidemiologic considerations will be addressed first, followed by some discussion of the importance of biologic/histologic types of melanoma. The microscopic evaluation and "histologic microstage" will serve as a basis for the final discussion of the therapeutic implications of the clinical and histologic evaluation of the patient with primary malignant melanoma.

PRECURSORS AND EPIDEMIOLOGIC CONSIDERATIONS

In the course of this discussion, we will be referring to "tumor progression". Although the term implies inevitable steps along a pathway, it should be understood that any individual lesion may 1) progress along the steps, 2) persist unchanged for long periods of time at any step or 3) regress, also at any stage. The steps begin with the benign tumor of melanocytes — — the melanocytic nevus or mole— through more disorderly nevi (the clinically atypical and histologically dysplastic nevus). The more controversial terms of atypical proliferations and in situ melanomas precede deeply invasive tumor. This sequence (Fig. 1) has been proposed and promoted by Wallace Clark and his co-workers.[7] It is based not only on the ex-

perimental models of Foulds[8] and others,[9] but also on the more recent work of Vogelstein et al, using the neoplastic transformation of the colonic mucosa.[10]

It is difficult to discuss the early, precursor lesions of melanoma without knowledge of the epidemiology of the disease. There is increasing evidence that individuals with light skin, born and raised in areas of high sunlight exposure, have not only increased numbers of moles, but also an increased incidence of melanoma. Emigration data from Ireland to Australia, from Europe to Israel, and from the northern parts of the U.S.A. to the southern parts, suggest that the sunlight exposure prior to the age of 18 may be a significant factor in the eventual development of melanoma.[11,12] Two important factors are at play: 1) The ability to tan: Children who tan poorly and experience

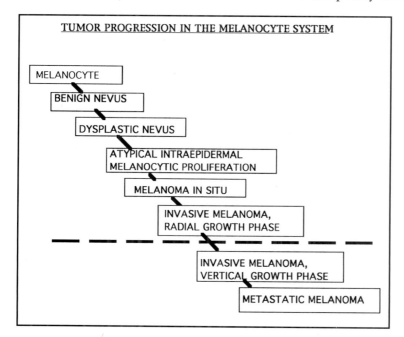

Fig. 1. Sequence of tumor progression in the melanocyte system adapted from Clark et al[7] and Vogelstein.[10] The line between radial and vertical growth separates curable from potentially uncurable neoplasia.

severe sunburns have increased numbers of moles and a higher incidence of adult melanoma. Children who tan easily do not have either an increase in their incidence of melanoma in later life or an increase in numbers of moles, in spite of early childhood sun exposure. 2) Genetic Factors: There seem to be familial tendencies for not only skin type, but the ability to form melanocytic nevi, and in turn, dysplastic nevi. In the subset of families with strong penetrance of atypical (dysplastic) nevi and a high incidence of malignant melanoma, genetic factors can play a dominant role.

ULTRAVIOLET EXPOSURE

The strongest association for the development of melanoma is that of fair-skinned people living in latitudes nearest the equator. Growing up in sunny latitudes, the inability to tan (sun sensitivity) and a history of severe sunburns in childhood all seem to play an important role in the relative risks for developing melanoma in adult life. Although there are some notable exceptions to the association of melanoma with prior UV exposure, 98% of melanomas from the general body skin occur in adult whites. Melanoma is a rare condition in the prepubertal child, with an instance of 0.1/100,000 (one in a million).

The incidence of melanoma from mucosal surfaces as well as palmar, plantar and subungual sites appears to be the same in all ethnic groups.[13] It has sometimes been implied that dark-skinned individuals have a higher incidence of melanoma from acral sites, but this is only in relation to the very few numbers of general body skin melanomas in these populations.

Relationship of Nevi to Melanoma

Melanocytic nevi are very common on the cutaneous surfaces. They are best thought of as benign tumors of the pigment cells. They are in general orderly and confined, both clinically and histologically. They are subclassified as (1) congenital and (2) acquired.

(1) Congenital nevi are defined clinically as those pigmented lesions present and apparent at or near birth. In studies of neonatal skin, 1–2% of newborns have pigmented nevi at birth.[14,15] The majority of these are solitary and small. Only about 1/20,000 have an intermediate size greater than 9.0 cm and perhaps one in half a million has a so-called giant or garment-sized nevus.[15] Often giant nevi are associated with multiple smaller congenital nevi around the large nevus and in the remaining cutaneous surfaces. Congenital nevi appear to be developmental defects arising early in embryologic life as witnessed by those arising on the face, showing evidence of nevus cells in both upper and lower eyelids, suggesting distribution of these cells prior to the separation of the eyelids in embryonic life.

Large congenital nevi are thought to have a 5–8% lifetime incidence of developing malignant melanoma. Some of the malignancies arise within the first few years of life, but such cases are almost reportably rare.[6] The incidence of malignant change in smaller congenital nevi is not yet known, but it is clear that some adult cutaneous melanomas arise in relation to both congenital and acquired melanocytic nevi.[17,18]

The congenital nevus seems to grow only relative to the body site, remaining relatively stable in appearance throughout life. Approximately 5% may undergo some lightening in color or even changes of partial or complete regression, occasionally with the development of a halo surrounding the lesion.

(2) Acquired melanocytic nevi: Nevi or moles which arise during childhood between the years of 3 and 6 are generally termed acquired nevi. Such nevi begin as small pigmented dots, gradually increasing to 4–6 mm. They tend to be uniform, round or oval and vary in color from flesh-colored to light or dark brown. They may undergo growth spurts during puberty or pregnancy. New nevi may be expected to develop up to perhaps the age of 40. They tend to stabilize following slight elevation and in later adult life become pale, flattened and often regress entirely. The numbers of acquired nevi seem to be directly related to the risk of developing melanoma.[19,20]

Studies of mole counts in control populations indicate that patients with melanoma have a higher overall number of melanocytic nevi than control individuals.[19] The total number of nevi appears to be a major risk factor for melanoma.[20] The relative risk of individuals having fewer than 25 moles is approximately 1.5 times the normal population, while those with more than 100 moles have a risk of approximately 10 times. Melanoma patients have 2–3 times as many normal nevi as the matched controls.[20,21] Patients with large numbers of nevi also seem to be those that have the clinically and histologically disordered nevus termed atypical mole or dysplastic nevus.

Dysplastic nevi have had a short but tumultuous career. They were described originally by both Clark and Lynch in 1978 in families with large numbers of unusual moles and a high incidence of malignant melanoma.[22,23] By 1980 it was recognized that melanoma patients in general, without a family history, also had disorderly nevi similar to those seen in the familial dysplastic nevus syndrome. These were tentatively termed sporadic dysplastic nevi.[24] Clinical-pathologic studies of smaller nevi gradually increased the diagnostic accuracy,[25] but it quickly became apparent that the criteria were still ill-defined. There is a spectrum from the common acquired benign nevus through the degrees of histologic dysplasia which have been defined as i) low grade and ii) severe[26] with regard to those lesions which are suspicious for melanoma. The relative risk of melanoma varies not only with the family history of unusual moles and melanoma, but also with the numbers of such nevi. Families with two or more members having melanoma and an affected child having dysplastic nevi have one of the highest risks of melanoma yet identified.[27] It is thought that such an affected individual (analogous to the affected member with familial polyposis of the colon) will have virtually 100% lifetime chance of developing the neoplasm. Of great interest, however, is the fact that siblings within a family of hereditary moles and melanoma who do not have the phenotypic expression of moles, have almost no risk for the development of the disease.[28]

It seems clear that there are many more individuals in the general population with dysplastic nevi of the so-called sporadic type than the several hundred hereditary melanoma kindreds which are known. The incidence of clinical atypical (dysplastic) moles varies from 5% to 50%.[29,30]

Of perhaps greatest importance are the studies indicating that follow-up of patients with these known risk factors (sunlight and precursor moles), with appropriate education and regular examinations of the cutaneous surfaces, can reduce the incidence of serious second lesions by picking up early, curable changes in benign or dysplastic moles, as well as new lesions from the intervening clinically normal skin.[31] In summary, (Fig. 2) moles, dysplastic moles and sun-sensitive skin with a relatively high childhood exposure to ultraviolet radiation, seem to be the main factors at the present time related to the risk of developing melanoma.

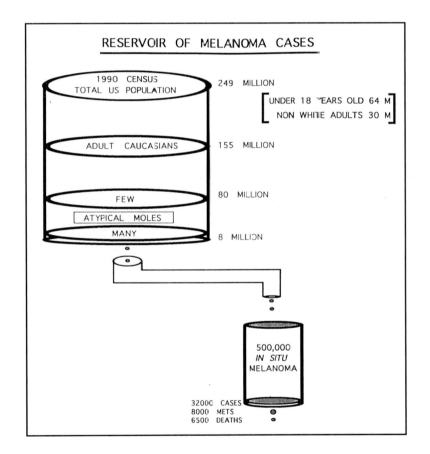

Fig. 2. Reservoir of cutaneous melanoma in the United States. These estimates of patients at risk can be helpful for public health planning. Because of the rarity of tumors in children less than 15 years of age or in people of pigment, the first major decrease in the reservoir is to the level of adult Caucasians. Patients with moles and/or atypical moles can be estimated to number from 8 to 80 million, of which 0.5 million could harbor melanoma in situ. The 32,000 annual diagnoses of invasive melanoma comes from this group, and in turn those with metastasis come from the invasive group and deaths come from the metastasis group (adapted from ref 30).

BIOLOGIC/HISTOGENETIC TUMOR TYPES

PRIMARY CUTANEOUS MALIGNANT MELANOMAS

Prior to 1969 primary cutaneous malignant melanoma was not subclassified as to histogenetic type. Melanomas generally were only identified as late, deep lesions, with an overall survival rate of less than 50%. As a result of Clark's original model of histogenetic types,[3] it was recognized that melanoma could be classified into subtypes which could be identified both clinically and histologically. Clark proposed a) Superficial spreading malignant melanoma b) nodular melanoma and c) lentigo maligna melanoma as useful histogenetic types. The fourth type, currently identified as acral lentiginous (palmar/plantar) melanoma was described later.[32]

Superficial Spreading Malignant Melanoma

The most common form of melanoma begins with a period of superficial growth across the surface of the skin, extending radially out from a theoretic center and only later developing deep invasion. This pattern of growth was called superficial spreading malignant melanoma (SSM) and accounts for more than two-thirds of the cutaneous melanomas in Caucasians. It can be found in any area of the body, but is common on the upper back of men and women and the lower extremities of women. (Fig. 3)

Clinically, patients report a change in a pre-existing pigmented lesion, in a wide range of approximately 20–80%.[33]

Histologically there is a similar range,[33] but in the UCSF experience, superficial spreading melanoma is associated with a recognizable associated nevus in approximately half the cases, somewhat greater in thinner tumors and less commonly in thicker tumors.[18] The clinical lesion of SSM is described as irregular in outline, irregular in pigmentation, and generally greater than 6–8 mm in diameter. The diagnostic accuracy of melanoma by clinicians seems to be approximately 60%,[34] suggesting there is room for improvement in the assessment, index of suspicion and criteria used in making the diagnosis of melanoma.

Radial Growth Phase: The radial growth phase (RGP) constitutes the initial proliferation in the malignant transformation of all types of melanoma except the nodular type. It is essentially defined as in situ and/or microinvasive tumor, in which no dominant clone of vertical growth has evolved. It is commonly associated with a dense cellular host response and appears to be virtually 100% curable with simple local excision. Regression, which is seen in about one-quarter of SSM, occurs almost exclusively within the radial growth phase, and when extensive, may be of prognostic importance.[35]

Fig. 3. Incidence of melanoma by sex and body sites at the Mt Zion/UCSF Melanoma Clinic. The clinic has accumulated a data base of 3750 prospectively entered patients since 1971. The 1753 cases presenting in clinical stage 1 SSM or NM are charted. Fig.3a. Lesions in men by eight body sites. Note the highest number in the upper back. Fig 3b. Lesions in women by eight body sites. Note the high incidence in the extremities, both upper and lower. The upper back in women is also an area of relatively high incidence.

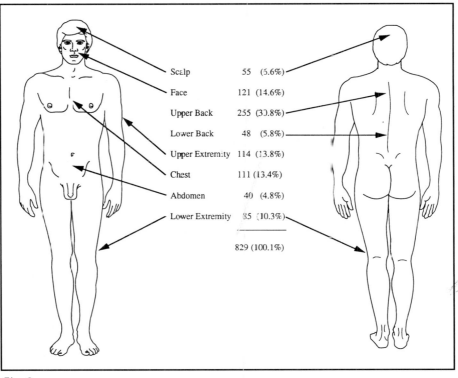

Scalp   55   (5.6%)
Face   121 (14.6%)
Upper Back   255 (30.8%)
Lower Back   48   (5.8%)
Upper Extremity 114 (13.8%)
Chest   111 (13.4%)
Abdomen   40   (4.8%)
Lower Extremity   85 (10.3%)
                 ─────────────
                 829 (100.1%)

Fig. 3a.

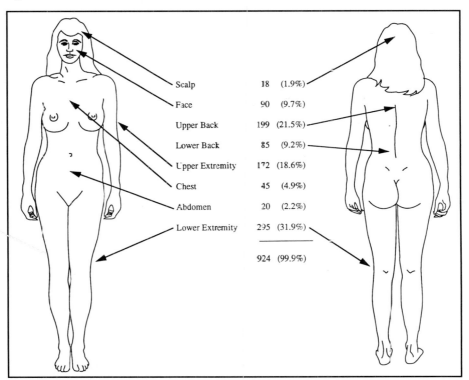

Scalp   18   (1.9%)
Face   90   (9.7%)
Upper Back   199 (21.5%)
Lower Back   85   (9.2%)
Upper Extremity 172 (18.6%)
Chest   45   (4.9%)
Abdomen   20   (2.2%)
Lower Extremity 295 (31.9%)
                 ─────────────
                 924 (99.9%)

Fig. 3b.

Vertical Growth Phase: The vertical growth phase (VGP) is identified clinically as a nodule arising de novo or within a macular or plaque-like, pigmented lesion and may be non-pigmented. Histologically it is a distinct population of cells, often without cellular host response, growing as an expansile sphere or sheet of cells. Mitotic figures and nuclear pleomorphism characterize these neoplastic cells. The deeper the invasion in terms of either anatomic levels[3] or tumor thickness in millimeters,[4] the more likely the tumor is to metastasize and ultimately kill the patient. Tumor thickness is probably the strongest histologic determinant of prognosis, especially in thicker tumors. In thin tumors less than 1.1 mm in tumor thickness there is evidence that the anatomic level of invasion as described by Clark is of prognostic importance.[36] In tumors greater than 1.1 mm in thickness, the measurement of tumor thickness in millimeters becomes dominant over level of invasion. Other important histologic microstage factors include mitotic index (numbers of mitotic figures per mm[2] in the vertical growth), regression (presence or absence of regression, as well as the percent of surface area involved), and the degree of cellular host response (also called tumor infiltrating lymphocytes). The concept of clinical and histologic differences between radial and vertical growth in melanoma has been summarized by Clark et al.[37]

Nodular Melanomas

Nodular melanomas can be thought of as the vertical growth phase without an associated RGP. Clinically, these lesions are more difficult to diagnose, as nodular melanoma may be verrucous and appear similar to warts, may be amelanotic and mimic hemangiomas, or may be uniformly pigmented and be confused with normal moles. Of interest is the fact that patients are more likely to notice changes in nodular melanoma than are physicians.[38] It is commonly thought that both SSM and nodular melanomas are similar in their evolution and, when corrected for tumor thickness, seem to have the same prognosis. It is not entirely clear whether other subtypes (LMM, ALM) have equal prognosis when corrected for tumor thickness. Amelanotic melanoma has a reputation for aggressive behavior, probably because it becomes deeply invasive prior to definitive diagnosis. SSM and nodular melanoma account for perhaps 85% of cutaneous melanoma in Caucasians.

Lentigo Maligna Melanoma

Lentigo maligna melanoma (LMM) arises from a slowly evolving macular pigmented lesion on sun-damaged skin. LMM was noted around the turn of the century by Jonathan Hutchinson and has been termed Hutchinson's melanotic freckle (HMF). It may enlarge to involve a large area of the face and extend over mucosal surfaces of the eye and/or mouth. The macular lesion shows irregular pigmentation and may have areas of regression. It is currently thought to be a) a precursor lesion, and/or b) the in situ or radial growth phase of this type of melanoma. It is probably both. Perhaps only 5–8% of lentigo malignas evolve to LMM.[39] The nodule arising in LM becomes the vertical growth and may only develop after many years of radial growth with or without therapy. It is difficult to determine with certainty whether the vertical growth of

LMM is equal in biologic behavior to that of nodular and SSM, as tumors of the face seem to have a relatively favorable prognosis,[40] and so one must compare sex and location as well as tumors of equal thickness when evaluating these tumor types. Some lentigo maligna melanomas have either desmoplastic or neurotrophic components, which affect both their rate of local recurrence, as well as their ultimate prognosis. The therapy of LMM at the Mt Zion/UCSF Melanoma Clinic is usually to excise the macular component (whenever possible) with relatively narrow margins of about 5 mm and follow the area closely. The therapy of desmoplastic/neurotrophic melanoma associated with LMM should be directed to the deep margin because of the tendency of this type to recur locally.

LMM seems to be epidemiologically more closely related to the non-melanoma skin cancers than the group of SSM and nodular melanomas. LMM occurs on sun-damaged skin, generally with an older average age. It has an age-related incidence roughly corresponding to actinic keratosis, squamous cell carcinoma and basal cell carcinoma.

Acral and Mucosal Lentiginous Melanoma

Melanomas arising in palms, soles and subungual regions have a distinctive radial growth phase, which is histologically lentiginous.[32] The radial growth phase of these, as well as mucosal lesions, may be varied in pigmentation, but appears macular. The vertical growth may be pigmented or non-pigmented, as in the case of SSM and nodular.

It has been questioned by Ackerman as to whether it is useful to separate histogenetic types [41] It is of course less challenging merely to make the diagnosis of "malignant melanoma," without attempting to subclassify the process. When one examines the epidemiologic, therapeutic and prognostic differences, however, it remains important to identify subtypes of melanoma. ALM, LMM and MLM are good examples of this.

The incidence of acral and mucosal lentiginous melanomas seems to be the same in all races.[13] ALM is not a common tumor, representing approximately 1–2% of all melanomas. This incidence is remarkably different from SSM/nodular melanomas, which appears to be almost exclusively a disease of white skin. The ALM arising in palms, soles and subungual regions is somewhat more difficult to estimate prognosis based on tumor thickness, although the disease appears to be aggressive in both men and women. In Clark's prognostic model of 1989,[42] acral lesions were classified with truncal lesions to distinguish them from the better prognosis of extremity lesions. The histologic features of ALM include a so-called lentiginous growth of individual melanocytes as single cells and small nests along the dermal-epidermal junction, often with a closely applied lymphocytic host response. The lymphocytes in this variant commonly cross the dermal-epidermal junction and surround individual cells in a rosette. This type of cellular host response is not common in cutaneous SSM and nodular tumors. It is occasionally seen in LMM. Extension down eccrine sweat glands, even to the level of the sweat coil, is common and should be looked for in the histologic specimen. The Clark levels of invasion such as papillary dermis (Level

II) or papillary reticular dermis interface (Level III) are not anatomically identifiable in normal subungual and in most areas of plantar skin. Therefore, the Clark levels are not applicable to these tumors. It is well-known that thin tumors in acral sites may present as metastatic melanoma. In general, however, thicker tumors have a worse prognosis than thinner tumors, as in the general body skin.

Primary Melanoma, Unusual Subtypes

The four major melanomas described above account for approximately 98% of cutaneous melanoma in people. A few unusual variants exist. Some of these have features which require a special approach to their therapy

Desmoplastic/Neurotrophic Melanoma

Melanomas whose vertical growth is associated with desmoplastic collagen may arise with or without a surface pigmented lesion.[43] Most commonly, desmoplastic melanoma (DMM) is seen in association with a lentigo maligna type macular pigmentation, but desmoplastic melanoma may also arise as a firm, cutaneous nodule lacking any distinctive features and often partially and/or superficially biopsied as dermatofibroma or scar. Unless the diagnosis is suspected and the biopsy is deep enough, the diagnosis may be missed, especially in lesions where the desmoplastic element predominates over tumor cells. Lymphocytic host response is commonly sparse. DMM may exhibit variable amounts of perineural extension. Where that pattern of growth is predominant, Reed and others have termed such lesions neurotrophic melanoma.[44] Both desmo-plasia and neurotrophism are important histologic findings, as they suggest tumors which will be prone to local recurrence. Deep local excision is advised. Desmoplastic melanoma in the head and neck region is more difficult to treat than truncal sites because of the numerous nerve trunks and extension into vital areas.

Mucosal (Lentiginous) Melanoma

Mucosal melanoma, sometimes termed mucosal lentiginous melanoma (MLM), has many features in common with ALM. Both have a lentiginous macular component to the radial growth phase along the dermal-epidermal junction. Both arise in areas of the body where the anatomic Clark levels are not uniformly present. Both seem somewhat more capricious in their behavior than reflected by tumor thickness alone, as both can metastasize when the tumor thickness is in a range which would be lower risk on the general body skin. Finally both present special problems in therapy based on their unique anatomic sites. MLM arises in oral and genital mucosal sites. Their poorer prognosis is often attributed to late diagnosis from sites which are hidden such as paranasal sinuses or perianal mucosa. In a neoplasm where surgery is the primary therapeutic tool, MLM represents a special challenge. Unlike ALM, where isolated heated limb perfusion can be an alternate approach to some difficult lesions, MLM is often difficult to control.

Melanoma Arising in Giant Congenital Nevus

In the neonatal period, small nodules of epithelioid melanocytes may be seen, including mitotic figures, which may enlarge, persist or regress in the neonatal period.[37] These lesions have sometimes been termed hyperplastic nodules and may be under some hormonal stimulus, which allows them to involute in later childhood. Larger, more rapidly growing lesions in association with congenital nevi, however, may represent malignant melanoma. Such tumors may have a neuroid or even pleomorphic appearance, with Schwannian or other primitive mesenchymal tissue forms reflected in the neoplasm. Mitotic activity is thought to be of prognostic importance.[16] The biologic behavior is variable, as some large tumors present at birth which are excised seem to be associated with a favorable prognosis, whereas other smaller nodules in the range of 5–10 mm which arise in the same time period may demonstrate widespread metastases.

Malignant Blue Nevus

On occasion, lesions which have a precursor blue nevus which may be atypical or large can undergo what appears to be malignant transformation with areas of necrosis and mitotic activity. Malignant blue nevus is generally defined by its biologic behavior of local recurrence and spread, rather than identifiable histologic features in the primary neoplasm.[37]

Verrucous Melanoma

Verrucous melanoma is best considered as a variant of SSM in which there is a reactive proliferation of the epidermis. In his original classification, Clark included verrucous melanoma as a separate variant which comprised about 10% of cases. Later these were included with SSM. Histologically they are not difficult to diagnose, although there is epidermal verrucous hyperplasia. Clinically, however, they may mimic seborrheic keratoses or warts because of the verrucous surface.

Melanoma of Soft Parts (Clear Cell Sarcoma)

Malignant melanoma of soft parts, formerly called clear cell sarcoma, is now identified as a variant of melanoma.[45] It occurs in young adults with a median age of 27 years, but may be seen in both children and older individuals. It is somewhat more common in women than in men, and may be seen both in Blacks and Asians. Melanoma of soft parts may begin as slowly growing tumor masses around the foot, ankle, knee or elbow areas. The prognosis is poor, as they metastasize readily to lungs. The tumor is made up of fascicles of large clear cells, which are S-100 protein positive in the majority of instances and may contain melanin pigment by the routine Fontana method. Premelanosomes may be seen in specimens prepared for electron microscopy.[46]

Minimum Deviation Melanoma

The term "minimum deviation" originally seemed to imply a lesion resembling a nevus — a "well-differentiated" melanoma. Over time, however, the concept seemed to evolve to include what seemed to be a broad range of types, such as the spindle cell variant. It does not seem to be a useful term until is is more clearly defined.[37]

METASTATIC MELANOMA

Once a melanoma has been demonstrated to have the capacity to metastasize, the prognosis is altered. The various types of metastasis, however, must be carefully defined. It is often the case in the literature on this subject that the term "recurrence" is used loosely. It is unclear whether the recurrence being discussed is local, regional or distant (systemic). Even when recurrence is called "local" it could refer to intraepidermal "persistent" disease as a result of inadequate therapy to the original lesion or "recurrent" disease which is actually a local satellite or metastasis. Persistent disease should not alter the prognosis in a way different from that of the primary. Recurrent disease is a reflection of the biology of the tumor. Local or regional satellites may or may not be associated with distant metastases. Metastases to regional lymph nodes (Clinical stage 2 disease by most staging systems) is usually thought to be associated with a 40% five-year survival. Distant metastases have a survival of approximately 5–7% at five years.[1] Hopefully some of the newer biologic therapies can improve these figures.

THE CONCEPT OF TUMOR PROGRESSION

If melanoma remained a localized tumor growth as in the case of basal cell carcinoma, it would be of little threat to the patient's life. The ability of such tumors to metastasize is the primary reason to learn to remove the earliest changing pigmented lesion. The concept of tumor progression is that of a spectrum which ends in a neoplasm capable of metastasis. We have traced in this chapter the progression from a benign tumor (melanocytic nevus) to a disorderly tumor (the dysplastic nevus), through in situ and microinvasive tumor (radial growth phase), to the vertical growth phase. Time is needed to evolve through these steps, and it is clear from the work in colon cancer that numerous regulated steps of oncogene activation and tumor suppressor gene deregulation occur, which allow for progressive steps. It is presumed that tumor cells escape from the local site at an early point in vertical growth phase and appear in the general circulation. The fascinating work of Fidler and his co-workers suggests that metastatic melanoma is also regulated.[9] They have found that injection of melanoma cells in the lower extremity of an experimental animal resulting in metastases in various organs can be identified as site-specific metastases. If, for example, the pulmonary metastases are removed and placed in a syngeneic animal, the next generation of tumors has a high likelihood of pulmonary spread. If this generation has its pulmonary nodule again placed in a syngeneic animal, the tumors will spread only to the lung. The concept of an organ-specific metastases implies a degree of regulation, and regulation implies something which can be studied, understood, and perhaps deregulated. Clinically one sees individuals with solitary or single organ involvement and occasionally surgical removal of such lesions results in long survival. Unfortunately, more commonly one sees multi-organ involvement with spread to brain, lungs, liver or bone all involved prior to death. The process of metastasis to lymph nodes raises enormous and as yet unsolved questions related to elective lymph node dissection. This is based in part on the fact that tumors may go through a stage where they are capable only of growth within lymph nodes. Removal of those nodes at such a time could result in clinical survival.

If the nodes are not removed, it is possible the tumor could modulate at the regional site, distributing tumor cells which could be capable of growth in other organs. The process of circulation of tumor cells throughout the body and growth in distant sites is complex and includes exposure to numerous environments where the host defenses can play an active role.

The same relationship of tumor progression to metastases can be found in the radial growth phase/vertical growth phase tumors. In the RGP it seems that the melanoma, despite its microinvasion through the basement membrane of the epidermis, has not yet learned to grow in other than the local environment. Thin VGP tumors have a low incidence of metastasis, but are still occasionally capable of spread. Thicker tumors have increasingly higher incidence of regional and distant spread.

Some tumors, despite deep invasion and factors which seem to make distant spread inevitable, still are associated with a favorable prognosis. Recent studies have shown favorable prognosis in deeply invasive tumors.[47] Perhaps such tumors have only learned to grow locally, despite their bulk.

MICROSTAGE EVALUATION

THE PATHOLOGY REPORT

Histologic evaluation of the primary melanoma is an important factor in establishing prognosis for the individual patient. Many of the factors evaluated help to determine therapy. Re-excision margins, depth of the re-excision specimen and elective lymph node dissection can be influenced by the histologic microstage evaluation. Other factors help to evaluate the likelihood of regional or distant spread, and finally, the microstage measurements in conjunction with the location of the tumor and the sex and age of the patient, are currently the best factors for assessing prognosis.

The Pathology Specimen

Because of the importance of the pathologic microstage in estimating prognosis and planning therapy, the specimen sent to the pathologist for evaluation should be taken with care. The ideal specimen is a narrow but complete excision of the suspicious pigment lesion.[48] Although this is emphasized in many textbooks, it is often neglected in the haste to make a diagnosis with shave, punch or other partial biopsies. Misdiagnoses and inappropriate therapies have resulted from such inadequate biopsies. Therapy should not be planned on partial biopsies.

If an adequate specimen is received and processed appropriately by the pathologist, the pathology report should allow the clinician to estimate prognosis and plan therapy. The report should include the following:

a) Histogenetic type.
b) Level of invasion.
c) Tumor thickness in millimeters.
d) Mitotic rate, and
e) Lymphocytic host response evaluation.

Figure 4 shows Clark's levels and Breslow's thickness in normal skin and melanoma. The basal cell layer marks the

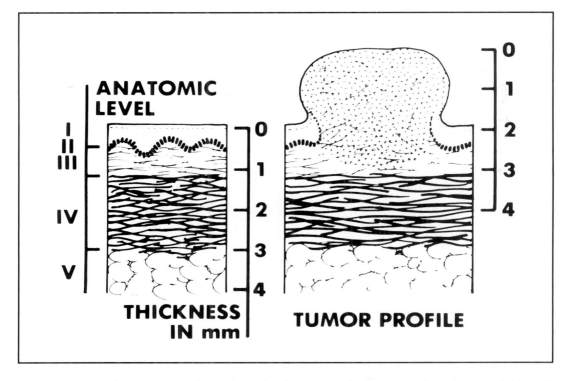

Fig. 4. Diagram of anatomic levels (Clark) and millimeters of thickness (Breslow) in normal skin (left) and in a typical tumor profile (right). Tumor thickness in millimeters helped to explain the problem of poor survival with thick, protuberant tumors whose apparent level was not deep.

margin of level I. Level II is within the papillary dermis, and level III extends to the papillary dermis. Level IV dips into the reticular dermis, and level V expands into the subcutaneous fat.

Other factors which may be helpful and in some instances are strong prognostic factors include:

f) Regression.
g) Ulceration.
h) Vascular invasion.
i) Microsatellites.

Finally, some evaluation of the presence of a precursor lesion, although it is not certain that it affects survival, is useful in ultimately following the patient.

CLINICAL FACTORS OF PROGNOSTIC IMPORTANCE

Gender

It has been commonly demonstrated that women survive melanoma better than men, even when stratified for tumor thickness.[42] This is especially true in tumors less than 1.7 mm in thickness. In thicker tumors the survival benefit is similar between the sexes.

Location

Malignant melanoma of the extremities is associated with a better survival than those on the trunk or axial skeleton.[42] When subsites are examined there appear to be subtle differences. For example, in the Mt Zion/UCSF Melanoma Center, chest and abdomen have markedly different survivals between men and women, but the numbers are small and meta-analysis would be needed between data bases to make a significant analysis. In the head and neck, however, studies show a difference between scalp and face, with scalp having a worse prognosis. Further subsite differences will soon be available as large data bases with long follow up are now beginning to have sufficient numbers of patients to make separate subsite analysis.

Age

Younger patients survive longer than older patients, even in multifactorial analyses which seem to correct for thickness. This seems to be true in Clinical Stages I, II or III.[49] It is true, however, that younger patients have thinner tumors and this question may need re-examination. Currently older men with scalp lesions seem to be the most rapidly increasing incidence, whereas in the previous decade it was lower extremity lesions in women.

SUMMARY

Although much has been learned about the natural history of malignant melanoma as a neoplasm, much remains to be done. Two important considerations should be addressed:

1) Public and physician education: As the general public begins to assume responsibility for its health, more education of risk groups is an important goal. However, it is still true that too many physicians fail to make a cutaneous examination a part of the primary care or annual physical examination.

2) Therapy for late stage melanoma: Although current four-drug chemotherapies can achieve a greater than 50% response rate, the responses are seldom long-lasting. Experimental therapies are still disappointing, with a low but finite and even long-lasting response rate.

Much effort is and should be devoted to both of these considerations and hopefully some goals can be met to deal with this neoplasm which will prevent the death of young and productive individuals.

REFERENCES

1. Balch CM and Milton GW (eds) Cutaneous melanoma. Clinical management and treatment results worldwide. 2nd edition. Philadelphia: JB Lippincott Co, 1992.
2. Koh H.K. Cutaneous melanoma. N Engl J Med 1991; 325:171-82.
3. Clark WH, From L, Berdardino EA, Mihm MC. The histogenesis and biologic behavior of primary human malignant melanoma of the skin. Cancer Res 1969; 29:705-27.
4. Breslow A. Thickness, cross-sectional areas and depth of invasion in the prognosis of cutaneous melanoma. Ann Surg 1970; 172:902-8.
5. Blois MS, Sagebiel RW, Abarbanel RM et al. Malignant melanoma of the skin I. The association of tumor depth and type, and patient sex, age and site with survival. Cancer 1983 52:1330-41.
6. Clark WH. Tumor progression and the nature of cancer. Brit J Cancer 1991; 64:631-64.
7. Clark WH, Elder DE, Guerry D et al. A study of tumor progression: the precursor lesions of superficial spreading and nodular melanoma. Hum Pathol 1984; 15:1147-65.

8. Foulds L. Neoplastic Development. Vol 1. Academic Press, New York, 1969.

9. Fidler IJ. The Biology of Melanoma Metastases in Cutaneous Melanoma. 2nd Ed. In: Balch CM, Milton GW, Houghton AN et al, eds. Philadelphia: JB Lippincott Co, 1992; 112-29.

10. Fearon ER, Vogelstein B. A genetic model for colorectal tumorigenesis. Cell 1990; 61:759-67.

11. Cooke KR, Fraser J. Migration and death from malignant melanoma. Int J Cancer 1985; 36:175.

12. Holman CDJ, Mulroney CD, Armstrong BK. Epidemiology of pre-invasive and invasive malignant melanoma in Western Australia. Int J Cancer 1980; 25:317.

13. Elwood JM. Epidemiology and control of melanoma in white populations and in Japan. J Invest Dermatol 1989; 92 (Suppl):214-18.

14. Walton RG, Jacobs AH, Cox AJ. Pigmented lesions in newborn infants. Br J Dermatol 1976; 95:389.

15. Castilla EC, Da Graci Dutra M, Orioli-Parvoiras IM. Epidemiology of congenital pigmented nevi: I. Incidence rates and relativity frequencies. Br J Dermatol 1981; 104:307.

16. Hendrickson MR, Ross, JC. Neoplasms arising in congenital giant nevi: morphologic study of seven cases and a review of the literature. Am J Surg Pathol 1981; 5:109-35.

17. Rhodes AR, Sober A, Day CL et al. The malignant potential of small congenital nevocellular nevi: an estimate of association based on the histologic study of 234 primary cutaneous melanomas. Am Acad Derm 1982; 6:230-41.

18. Sagebiel RW. Melanocytic nevi in histologic association with primary cutaneous melanoma of superficial spreading and nodular types: Effect of tumor thickness. In Press, 1992

19. Holly EA, Kelly JW, Shpall SN, Chiu SH. Number of melanocytic nevi as a major risk factor for malignant melanoma. J Am Acad Dermatol 1987; 17:459-68.

20. Beral V, Evans S, Shaw H, Milton G. Cutaneous factors related to the risk of malignant melanoma. ?JOURNAL?1983; 109:165-72.

21. Augustsson, A. Melanocytic naevi, melanoma and sun xxposure. Acta Dermato-Venerol 1991, Suppl 166. Dept of Dermatology Thesis, University of Goteborg, Sweden.

22. Clark WH, Reimer RR, Greene MH et al. Origin of familial malignant melanoma from heritable melanocytic lesions. "The B-K mole syndrome." Arch Dermatol 1978; 114:732-8.

23. Lynch HT, Frichot BC III, Lynch JF. Familial atypical multiple mole-melanoma syndrome. J Med Genet 1978; 15:352.

24. Elder DE, Goldman LI, Goldman SC et al. Dysplastic nevus syndrome: a phenotypic association of sporadic cutaneous melanoma. Cancer 1980;46:1787-94.

25. Kelly JW, Crutcher WA, Sagebiel RW. Clinical diagnosis of dysplastic melanocytic nevi. A clinicopathologic correlation. J Am Acad Dermatol 1986; 14:1044-52.

26. Sagebiel RW. Diagnosis and management of premalignant melanocytic proliferations. Pathology 1985; 17:298-290.

27. Kraemer KH, Greene MH, Tarone R et al. Dysplastic Naevi and cutaneous melanoma risk [letter] Lancet ii 1983; 1076.

28. Tucker MA. Individuals at high risk of melanoma. In: Elwood JM, ed. Melanoma and Nevi: Incidence, Interrelationships and Implications. Karger (Basel) Pigment Cell: vol 9: 95-109, 1988-1990.

29. Piepkorn M, Meyer LJ, Goldgar D et al. The dysplastic melanocytic nevus: a prevalent lesion that correlates poorly with clinical phenotype. J Am Acad Dermatol 1989; 20:407-15.

30. Sagebiel RW. The dysplastic nevus. J Am Acad Dermatol 1989; 20:496-501.

31. Greene MH, Clark WH, Tucker MA et al. High risk of malignant melanoma in melanoma-prone families with dysplastic nevi. Ann Intern Med 1985; 102:458-65.

32. Reed RJ. New Concepts in surgical pathology of the skin. In: Hartman W, Kay S, Reed RJ, eds. Histopathology. New York: John Wiley and Sons, 1976;27.

33. Elder DE, Greene MH, Bondi EE, Clark WH Jr. Acquired melanocytic nevi and melanoma: The Dysplastic Nevus Syndrome. In: Ackerman AB, ed. Pathology of Malignant Melanoma. New York: Masson Publishing Co., 1981:185-216.

34. Grin CM, Kopf AW, Welkovich B et al. Accuracy in the clinical diagnosis of malignant melanoma. Arch Dermatol 1990; 126:763-6.

35. Sagebiel RW. Regression and other factors of prognostic interest in malignant melanoma. Arch Dermatol 1985; 121:1125-6.

36. Kelly JW, Sagebiel RW, Clyman S, Blois MS. Thin level IV malignant melanoma: a subset in which Level is the major prognostic indicator. Ann Surg 1985; 202: 98-103.

37. Clark WH Jr, Elder DE, Guerry D IV. Dysplastic nevi and malignant melanoma, Chpt 49 In: Farmer ER, Hood AF eds. Pathology of the Skin. Appleton & Lange, 1990:684-756.

38. Cassileth BR, Temoshok L, Frederick BE et al. Patient and physician delay in melanoma diagnosis. J Am Acad Dermatol 1988; 18: 591-8.

39. Weinstock MA, Sober AJ. The risk of progression of lentigo maligna to lentigo maligna melanoma. Br J Dermatol 1987; 116:303-10.

40. McGovern VJ, Shaw, HM, Milton GW, Farago GA. Is malignant melanoma arising in a Hutchinson's melanotic freckle a separate disease entity? Histopathology 1980; 4:235-242.

41. Ackerman AB. Malignant melanoma: A unifying concept. Hum Pathol 1980; 11:591-5.

42. Clark WH Jr, Elder DE, Guerry D IV et al. Model predicting survival in stage I melanoma based on tumor progression. J Natl Cancer Inst 1989; 81:1893-1904

43. Egbert BM, Kempson R, Sagebiel RW. Desmoplastic malignant melanoma. Cancer 1988; 62:2033-41.

44. Reed RJ, Leonard DD. Neurotrophic melanoma: A variant of desmoplastic melanoma. Am J Surg Pathol 1979; 3:301-11.

45. Sara AS, Evans HL, Benjamin RS. Malignant melanoma of soft parts (Clear Cell Sarcoma): a study of 17 cases with emphasis on prognostic factors. Cancer 1990; 65:367-74.

46. Bearman RM, Noe J, Kempson RL. Clear cell sarcoma with melanin pigment. Cancer 1975; 36:977-84.

47. Coit D, Sauven P, Brennan M. Prognosis of thick cutaneous melanoma of the trunk and extremity. Arch Surg 1990;125:322-6.

48. National Institutes of Health Concensus Conference on Early Malignant Melanoma, Jan 27-29, 1992. (In Press).

49. Balch CW, Seng-Jaw S, Shaw HM et al. An analysis of prognostic factors in 8500 patients with cutaneous melanoma. In: Cutaneous Melanoma. 2nd Ed. Philadelphia: JB Lippincott Co., 1992;165-87.

CHAPTER 2

EARLY DIAGNOSTIC APPROACHES FOR HUMAN MELANOMA

Lee S. Albert and Arthur J. Sober*

Early detection of melanoma is the key to cure. When a melanoma is detected at a thickness of less than 0.76 mm, five-year survival rate ranges from 93 to 100% in different centers.[1] If a melanoma is not detected until thickness is over 4 mm, then five-year survival is reduced to 30 to 67%.[1] (Table 1) In situ melanoma (totally confined to the epidermis) is considered 100% curable by surgical excision.

How can early detection of melanoma be achieved? One approach to early detection is education. Education requires teaching not only dermatologists and other health professionals, but also the general public, to identify early melanoma. If melanoma is to be excised as early as possible, to ensure probable cure, then it has to be suspected and recognized.

Table 1.

Tumor Thickness	Five- Year Survival
Less than 0.76 mm	93-100%
0.76-1.49 mm	50-100%
1.50-2.49 mm	50-84%
2.50-3.99 mm	50-77%
4.00 mm or more	30-67%

The data illustrate that early detection of melanoma, at a stage when thickness is reduced, can lead to increased survival. These figures represent 5-year survival after melanoma diagnosis; the ranges represent the experiences of twelve centers worldwide, with some centers reporting higher survival, and some reporting lower survival, at each thickness. This table is modified from Balch et al.[1]

*Prepared with partial support from the Marion Gardner Jackson Trust, Bank of Boston, Trustee.

Recognizing melanoma (Figs. 1-3) is not always easy. Abnormalities in a pigmented lesion which should raise suspicion for melanoma can be summarized using the convenient mnemonic A-B-C-D: Asymmetry of the lesion; irregularity of the Border with blending into the surrounding skin; Color abnormality (with variegated pigment and shades of pink, white, tan, or brown, or with any component of black); and large Diameter (most melanomas are greater than 5 mm in largest diameter).[2,3,4] The A-B-C-D mnemonic has been popularized in American public health campaigns; an alternative seven point checklist has proved useful in Scottish public health campaigns.[2,5] The seven point checklist includes three major signs of melanoma (change in size, change in shape, and change in color) and three minor signs (inflammation, crusting or bleeding, sensory change including itch, and diameter greater than or equal to 7 mm).[5] Another useful criterion is to look for any one pigmented lesion which is acting differently (marching out of step) from the rest of the patient's nevi. Patients need to know that any lesion (nevus or "mole") which is suspicious for melanoma based on these criteria should be evaluated immediately by a physician. The most common signs recognized in early melanoma are increase in size (width) and change in color (darkening, lightening, or introduction of other colors). Excellent informational pamphlets regarding melanoma, with useful illustrations, are available.[6]

DIFFERENTIAL DIAGNOSIS

Obviously, not all pigmented lesions which meet the above mentioned criteria ultimately will prove to be melanoma, and there may be a wide differential diagnosis.[3,4] Seborrheic keratoses (Fig. 4) are benign nonmelanocytic lesions which will often meet many of the above criteria: seborrheic keratoses tend to be asymmetric, to have irregular borders, to have a variety of colors (including dark brown or black), and to have large diameter. Sensory change (itching), bleeding, or growing is also common in seborrheic keratoses. Seborrheic keratoses differ from melanoma, however, because they have a "stuck-on" appearance; the entire seborrheic keratosis looks like it can be peeled off the surface without disturbing the underlying skin. Seborrheic keratoses also tend to have horn cysts, but these can be seen in melanocytic lesions as well, so horn cysts are unfortunately not always a useful discriminator.

Another nonmelanocytic lesion which can be confused with melanoma is the pigmented basal cell carcinoma which is similar to other types of basal cell carcinomas except for an increase in melanin content. Superficial spreading pigmented actinic keratoses (SPAK) may mimic lentigo maligna or lentigo maligna melanoma, especially when they occur on the face; SPAK's surface may be rougher to touch than that of lentigo maligna. Vascular lesions such as hemangiomas (Fig. 5), angiokeratomas (Fig. 6) and pyogenic granulomas may be red-black in color and some may ulcerate or bleed, mimicking melanoma. Dermatofibromas are firm dermal lesions attached to the cutaneous surface which are occasionally pigmented, sometimes raising suspicion of melanoma. The presence of the characteristic dimpling with lateral compression helps to suggest the correct diagnosis. Tinea nigra

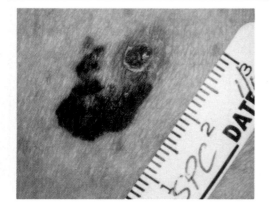

Fig. 1. Superficial spreading melanoma, level II, 0.51 mm. Note Asymmetry, Border irregularity, Color variegation, and large Diameter (the A-B-C-D characteristics).

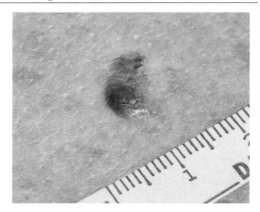

Fig. 2. Melanoma, level III, 1.2 mm. The A-B-C-D characteristics are evident.

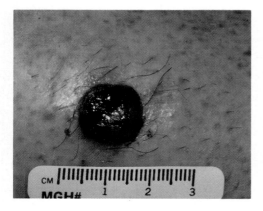

Fig. 3. Nodular melanoma, level IV, 3.8 mm. Although relatively symmetric and regularly bordered, this thicker more advanced melanoma has color com-ponents of red and black and a large diameter. The friable surface would likely lead to bleeding.

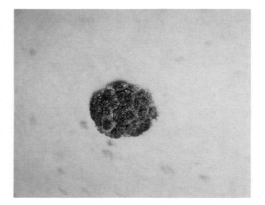

Fig. 4 .This seborrheic keratosis is large and dark colored, raising suspicion of melanoma. Its stuck-on appearance and horn cysts suggest the correct diagnosis.

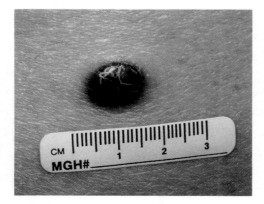

Fig. 5. This hemangioma is large and dark and may bleed, and looks similar to the nodular melanoma in Fig. 3. Biopsy may be required to make the correct diagnosis.

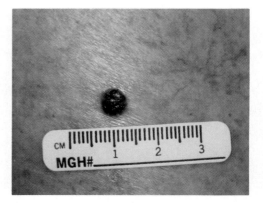

Fig. 6. This angiokeratoma, like other vascular lesions, may mimic melanoma.

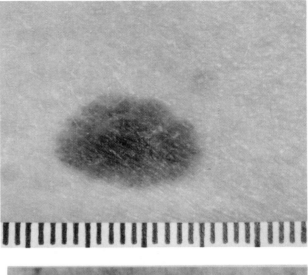

Fig. 7. This dysplastic nevus shares some of the A-B-C-D characteristics of melanoma, but to a lesser degree. Dysplastic nevi may be melanoma precursors as well as markers of individuals at increased risk for melanoma elsewhere on the skin.

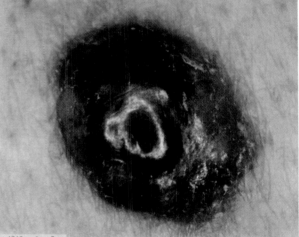

Fig. 8. Nodular melanoma. The Vanguard Imaging Ltd. prototype Digital ELMTM camera system was used to produce these images.

Fig. 8a shows the digital surface view without oil, and Fig. 8b shows the digital surface view with oil.

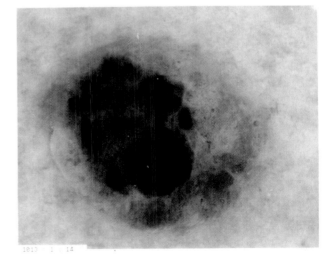

Note in Fig. 8b the prominent "milky way" or "veil," which corresponds to compact orthokeratosis and an increased granular layer, sometimes seen in melanoma. Copyright 1990, Vanguard Imaging Ltd. Images reprinted with permission from Kenet RO et al.[17]

is a superficial fungal infection which may be mistaken for acral lentiginous melanoma, but which should have a positive fungal potassium hydroxide preparation and culture. Subungual hematoma, usually induced by trauma, may be mistaken for subungual melanoma. Unlike melanoma, a subungual hematoma should clear with growth of the nail plate. Hutchinson's sign (hyperpigmentation of the adjacent cuticle) suggests melanoma rather than subungual hematoma, but is often absent even when melanoma is present.

The clinical differential diagnosis of melanoma includes not only nonmelanocytic lesions, but also a variety of melanocytic lesions. These include congenital nevi (which can be quite large and sometimes atypical appearing clinically), dysplastic nevi (which may share some of the atypical features of melanoma, but usually to a lesser degree) (Fig. 7), Spitz nevi (which are seen more commonly in children, but sometimes in adults), blue nevi (which may appear almost black because of the refraction of light by the dermal melanocytic proliferation), and solar lentigines (which can occasionally occur with a black starburst pattern).

Amelanotic nodular melanomas[7] and desmoplastic melanomas are real challenges to early diagnosis. These relatively rare variants are very difficult to diagnose because of lack of clinically apparent pigmentation which is a feature of most melanomas. These types usually can not be diagnosed at an early stage unless clinical suspicion is very high. Amelanotic nodular melanoma and desmoplastic melanoma can easily be mistaken for a nonmelanocytic neoplasm such as basal cell carcinoma, squamous cell carcinoma, Bowen's disease, or keratoacanthoma.

ACCURACY OF CLINICAL DIAGNOSIS

Even experienced dermatologists do not have 100% diagnostic accuracy when clinically assessing melanoma. Grin et al[8] reviewed clinical and pathologic diagnoses of biopsies and excisions from the Oncology Section of New York University's Skin and Cancer Unit. Over 10,000 specimens were submitted during the period 1955 through 1982. Primary melanoma was diagnosed clinically in 293 cases but confirmed histologically in only 214 (positive predictive value was 73%). On the other hand, 51 specimens which were histologically confirmed to be melanoma were not felt clinically to be melanoma (sensitivity was 80.8%). Nondermatologists are less able than dermatologists to diagnose melanoma and discriminate between melanoma and other types of pigmented lesions. Ramsay and Fox[9] showed pictures of typical dermatoses and skin neoplasms to dermatology residents and to primary care physicians in order to test their diagnostic acumen. All of the dermatologists recognized the pictures of a melanoma and of a seborrheic keratosis. In contrast, 88% of the primary care physicians recognized the slide of melanoma, and only 33% of the primary care physicians recognized the seborrheic keratosis. Similarly, Cassileth et al[10] showed pictures felt to be representative and characteristic of melanoma, dysplastic nevi and other lesions to dermatologists and to internists. Only 27% of dermatologists recognized six of six melanomas shown, and 71% recognized two of two dysplastic nevi shown. Among internists, 2% recognized all six melanomas, and 11% recognized both dysplastic nevi. This study's use of 35 mm color transparencies may have made diagnosis more difficult than direct clinical inspection. Still, the poor ability to identify melanoma demonstrated in this study suggests what most dermatologists have learned from their practices: that melanoma cannot always be recognized with certainty from its clinical appearance.

Andersen and Silvers[7] studied 13 clinically unsuspected melanomas that were diagnosed only by the pathologist. Eight of these were amelanotic and five were verrucous variants (hyperkeratotic). Incorrect clinical diagnoses by dermatologists had included basal cell carcinoma and seborrheic keratosis (four cases each), nevus (two cases), and Bowen's disease, keratoacanthoma, and verruca vulgaris (one case each).

EPILUMINESCENCE MICROSCOPY

How can physicians become better skilled at diagnosing melanomas and differentiating them from other pigmented lesions? In addition to education and experience, new tools and technologies may enhance the diagnostician's abilities. A simple 10x hand lens allows magnification to aid in the visualization of detail. Applying oil to the lesion may also be useful in altering the surface refractile properties of the lesion and allowing better visualization of such sub-surface characteristics as horn cysts and pigment patterns. The technique of epiluminescence microscopy[11-15] combines the benefits of magnification and oil to give a more accurate clinical diagnosis before resorting to biopsy. Pigment patterns can

be analyzed with the aid of immersion oil, a glass slide, and a magnifying stereomicroscope. The patterns observed have been named somewhat creatively, using terms such as "pigment network," "brown globules," "milky way," "black dots," and "pseudopods."[11] Each pattern appears to correspond with a particular histologic appearance seen on subsequent biopsy. The "pigment network," for instance, corresponds to pigmented rete ridges, and the "brown globules" correspond to nevomelanocytic nests in the papillary dermis. The "milky way" appearance corresponds to compact orthokeratosis and hypergranulosis of the epidermal keratinocytes which might be seen in melanoma. (Fig 8) Pehamberger et al[12] studied several thousand pigmented lesions using a binocular epiluminescence microscope (WILD M650, Wild Heerbrugg AG, Heerbrugg, Switzerland) which could obtain magnifications of up to 40x for clinical assessment. Analyzing pigment patterns, they noted differences between benign melanocytic lesions and malignant ones. Superficial spreading melanoma, for instance, often showed "black dots" at the periphery, corresponding to melanin in the stratum corneum, and "pseudopods" at the border, corresponding to confluent junctional nests. In order to test the abilities of such epiluminescence microscopy findings to improve diagnostic accuracy, Steiner et al[13] used the WILD M650 to analyze 318 small pigmented lesions which were considered clinically equivocal. All of the lesions were subsequently excised. They compared the diagnosis made with the epiluminescence microscope and the diagnosis made clinically without it, to see which corresponded better to the final histologic findings. Diagnoses with the epiluminescence microscope outperformed routine clinical diagnosis, with diagnostic accuracy of 85% compared to 61%. Thirty-nine of the lesions were invasive superficial spreading melanomas; the epiluminescence microscope detected 90% of these, compared to only 64% diagnosed without it. Seventy-five of the lesions were dysplastic nevi; the epiluminescence microscope recognized 82% of these, compared to only 60% recognized without it. An example of a currently available relatively inexpensive epiluminescence microscope is the Delta 10 dermatoscope, made by Heine USA in Cary, North Carolina. If preliminary experience with these devices can be confirmed in general usage, then a decreasing percentage of clinically equivocal lesions may need to be biopsied.

COMPUTER IMAGING

The use of computer technology may lead to future advances in melanoma detection.[16-20] Computer imaging can help to objectify the somewhat subjective impressions used by clinicians in deciding whether or not a lesion is suspicious for melanoma. The basic goal of computer imaging is simple: to represent a pigmented lesion as an array of numbers (digitizing), allowing quantitative analysis of the lesion. The computer imaging system divides the surface area of a pigmented lesion into a grid composed of hundreds or thousands of tiny squares. The computer can then represent the pigmented lesion as a series of numbers, each number corresponding to the amount of light reflected by the lesion in one small square. Color can be represented by assigning three values to each square, based on the amount

of red, green and blue light reflected. The computer can display the image of the lesion on a screen with each number converted into a picture element (pixel) of appropriate hue and intensity. The image can be permanently stored and compared with images of the same lesion at a later time to check for changes that might suggest malignancy. Moreover, the series of numbers representing the lesion can be subjected to analysis and to transformations designed to enhance contrast and differentiate between different types of lesions. The digital image can be transformed to eliminate background noise and to focus in on aspects such as border irregularity or color variegation. Data on images can be transferred by computer disk or modem for analysis at a distance from the acquisition site.

An imaging system developed by Vanguard Imaging in Cambridge, MA has been used at Massachusetts General Hospital. Interestingly, this system combines epiluminescence microscopy with digital imaging to produce images with very sharp detail and contrast from which "pseudopods" and "milky ways" can be read with ease.[16,17]

Green et al[18] used an IBM-compatible AT computer and 11 image analysis measurements to analyze pigmented lesions. They included such variables as fragmentation index and red, green and infrared variance (with "FRAG" corresponding to $4 \times pi \times area / perimeter^2$). "FRAG" would be 1 for a perfect circle, with progressively lower values occurring for increasingly irregular lesions. Analyzing 70 pigmented lesions, including 53 nevi and five melanomas, they achieved a 76% accurate classification with their system compared to less than 50% accuracy using clinical parameters without imaging.

Alternatively, Cascinelli et al[19] used two coupled IBM computers (7350/4561) to digitally represent the light transmitted by slides of different types of pigmented lesions. They then subjected the data to Fourier transformation. Fourier spectrum images were subsequently produced: melanoma produced an image described by them as a"galaxy;" benign nevus produced a "stain," and seborrheic keratosis produced a "cross."

It should be noted that digital imaging can be applied not only to light reflected by a pigmented lesion but also to other characteristics. For instance, mapping reflection of sound waves by a lesion can produce an ultrasound image, while mapping proton characteristics within a lesion can produce an MRI image.[20-22] Both technologies are being studied for their value in assessing pigmented lesions.

One future use of digital imaging would be to store images of a patient's

Table 2. Epiluminescence Microscopy: Selected Terminology (modified from Bahmer FA et al[11] and Soyer HP et al[14])

	TERM	HISTOLOGY	DIAGNOSIS
1.	Pigment network	Elongated rete ridges with basal layer melanocytic hyperplasia	Melanocytic lesion (broadened in early melanoma)
2.	Black dots	Clumped melanin in stratum corneum	Melanoma
3.	Whitish veil (milky way)	Compact orthokeratosis, increased granular layer	Melanoma
4.	Maple leaf areas	Nodules of pigmented basaloid cells	Basal cell carcinoma
5.	Yellow-white dots	Horn cysts	Seborrheic keratosis
6.	Brown globules	Papillary dermal nests	Irregular in melanoma, regular in dermal nevus
7.	Pseudopods	Peripheral confluent junctional nests	Melanoma
8.	Red-blue areas	Dilated papillary vessels	Vascular lesion (e.g. hemangioma)

nevi in a computer database. Scanning the patient's nevi at subsequent visits, the computer might be able to determine which of the nevi had undergone change in regard to symmetry, border, color or diameter. Currently conventional photography is used by some dermatologists for much the same purpose, with Polaroid or 35 millimeter photographs of nevi filed for future comparison.[23] Digital imaging might allow quantitative comparisons as opposed to the qualitative comparisons permitted by conventional photography.

Digital imaging is still in its infancy, though, and no method has yet appeared that would allow perfect discrimination of benign and malignant lesions.[21] Digital imaging has a long way to go before it becomes a preferred method of deciding whether or not a lesion is melanoma. For now, in general, any lesion at all suspicious for melanoma should be excisionally biopsied whenever it is clinically feasible to do so.[24] Histology remains the gold standard for melanoma diagnosis.

SUMMARY

Unlike many other cancers, melanoma affects young persons disproportionately and is therefore a leading cause of premature death.[24] Most melanomas can be cured, when they are still thin, with simple excisional surgery. New and old techniques for early recognition of melanoma can save many years of life and prevent substantial morbidity and mortality.[24]

REFERENCES

1. Balch CM, Cascinelli N, Drzewiecki KT et al. A comparison of prognostic figures worldwide. In: Balch CM, Houghton AN, Milton GW, Sober AJ, Soong S (eds). Cutaneous Melanoma. 2nd ed. Philadelphia: JB Lippincott, 1992;194.

2. McGovern TW, Litaker MS. Clinical predictors of malignant pigmented lesions. A comparison of the Glasgow seven-point checklist and the American Cancer Society's ABCDs of Pigmented Lesions. J Dermatol Surg Oncol 1992; 18:22-6.

3. Fitzpatrick TB, Milton GW, Balch CM et al. Clinical characteristics. In Balch CM, Houghton AN, Milton GW, Sober AJ, Soong S, eds. Cutaneous Melanoma. 2nd ed. Philadelphia: JB Lippincott, 1992;229-30.

4. Friedman RJ, Rigel DS. The clinical features of malignant melanoma. Dermatol Clin 1985; 3:271-83.

5. MacKie RM. Clinical recognition of early invasive malignant melanoma. Looking for changes in size, shape and colour is successful. Br Med J 1990; 301:1005-6.

6. Grossman DJ. Public and professional educational materials on skin cancer. J Am Acad Dermatol 1989; 21:1012-18.

7. Andersen WK, Silvers DN. Melanoma? It can't be melanoma! A subset of melanomas that defies clinical recognition. JAMA 1991; 266:3463-5.

8. Grin CM, Kopf AW, Welkovich B et al. Accuracy in the clinical diagnosis of malignant melanoma. Arch Dermatol 1990; 126:763-6.

9. Ramsay DL, Fox AB. The ability of primary care physicians to recognize the common dermatoses. Arch Dermatol 1981; 117:620-2.

10. Cassileth BR, Clark WH Jr, Lusk EJ et al. How well do physicians recognize melanoma and other problem lesions. J Am Acad Dermatol 1986; 14:555-60.

11. Bahmer FA, Fritsch P, Kreusch J et al. Terminology in surface microscopy. Consensus meeting of the Committee on Analytical Morphology of the Arbeitsgemeinschaft Dermatologische Forschung, Hamburg, Federal Republic of

Germany, Nov. 17, 1989. J Am Acad Dermatol 1990; 23:1159-62.

12. Pehamberger H, Steiner A, Wolff K. In vivo epiluminescence microscopy of pigmented skin lesions. I. Pattern analysis of pigmented skin lesions. J Am Acad Dermatol 1987; 17:571-83.

13. Steiner A, Pehamberger H, Wolff K. In vivo epiluminescence microscopy of pigmented skin lesions II. Diagnosis of small pigmented skin lesions and early detection of malignant melanoma. J Am Acad Dermatol 1987; 17:584-91.

14. Soyer HP, Smolle J, Hodl S et al. Surface Microscopy. A new approach to the diagnosis of cutaneous pigmented tumors. Am J Dermatopathol 1989; 11:1-10.

15. MacKie RM. An aid to the preoperative assessment of pigmented lesions of the skin. Br J Dermatol 1971; 85:232-8.

16. Kenet RO, Kang S, Barnhill RL et al. Melanoma and melanoma precursors-pigment pattern characterization in vivo using computer-assisted epiluminescence microscopy (abstract). J Cutan Pathol 1990; 17:304

17. Kenet RO, Kang S, Barnhill RL et al. Differential diagnosis of melanocytic neoplasms in vivo using digital epiluminescence microscopy. An atlas (submitted for publication).

18. Green A, Martin N, McKenzie G et al. Computer image analysis of pigmented skin lesions. Melanoma Research 1991; 1:231-6.

19. Cascinelli N, Ferrario M, Tonelli T, Leo E. A possible new tool for clinical diagnosis of melanoma: The computer. J Am Acad Dermatol 1987; 16:361-7.

20. Perednia DA. Developing uses for digital imaging in the diagnosis and treatment of melanoma. Diagnosis and Treatment of Early Melanoma. NIH Consensus Development Conference. 1992; 87-90.

21. Perednia DA. What dermatologists should know about digital imaging. J Am Acad Dermatol 1991; 25:89-108.

22. Zemtsov A, Lorig R, Ng TC et al. Magnetic resonance imaging of cutaneous neoplasms: clinicopathologic correlation. J Dermatol Surg Oncol 1991; 17:416-22.

23. Ho VC, Milton GW, Sober AJ. Biopsy of melanoma. In: Balch CM, Houghton AN, Milton GW, Sober AJ, Soong S (eds): Cutaneous Melanoma. 2nd ed. Philadelphia: JB Lippincott, 1992;265-8.

24. Albert VA, Koh HK, Geller AC et al. Years of potential life lost: another indicator of the impact of cutaneous malignant melanoma on society. J Am Acad Dermatol 1990;23:308-10.

CHAPTER 3

SURGICAL TREATMENT OF PRIMARY MELANOMA

Stanley P.L. Leong

Microstaging of melanoma using Clark's level and Breslow's thickness is crucial in predicting its clinical outcome. The current surgical approach of melanoma, based on histologic diagnosis and microstaging,[8-13] has revolutionized the treatment of melanoma. Although the incidence of malignant melanoma is rising rapidly, doubling every 10 years, the overall mortality has increased slightly, indicating that a significant proportion of the melanoma being diagnosed is of the thin level and can be effectively treated by definitive surgical resection.[32,42,67] Based on the thickness of the primary melanoma, the re-excision margin can be tailored to individual patients rather than to the traditional approach of a 5 cm margin. Further, it is the general consensus that no elective lymph node dissection is required for thin melanoma less than 1 mm. For melanoma thicker than 1 mm, the role of elective lymph node dissection is still controversial. This chapter addresses the issues a surgeon will face in dealing with a patient with a newly-diagnosed melanoma.

DIAGNOSIS OF MELANOMA

When a cutaneous lesion or mole undergoes a change in size, color, shape, contour or sensation, it should be biopsied.[35] An excisional biopsy (Fig. 1) is usually done so that the entire lesion, including the subcutaneous fat, can be submitted to the pathologist for histologic diagnosis and microstaging, as it has been well established that microstaging is crucial in predicting the outcome of melanoma.[8-13] Traditional concerns that incision into a melanoma could result in a dissemination has not been substantiated by recent studies.[5,27,45,65] The survival of patients undergoing excisional biopsy showed no difference from those who had incisional

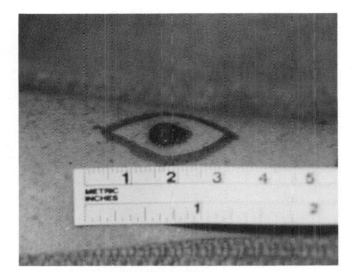

Figs. 1A-C. This is a 25-year-old Caucasian female who had a suspected elevated pigmented skin lesion in the left forearm.

Fig. 1A. An excisional biopsy was performed as shown here. A 2 mm margin was obtained with additional extension in the superior and inferior direction of the longitudinal elliptical incision.

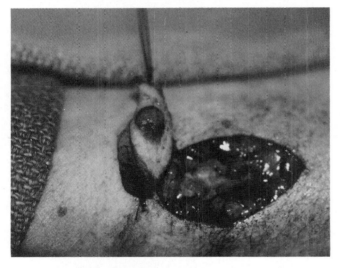

Fig. 1B. The lesion is shown to contain adequate amount of adipose tissue for microstaging. The specimen was labeled with stitches in situ for pathological orientation

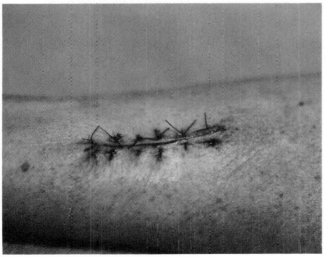

Fig. 1C. The wound was closed primarily. Final pathology showed nodular melanoma, Clark's level III and Breslow thickness 1.05 mm. As it is shown here, the superior and inferior margins are much more than 2 mm in order to have the wound closed in a cosmetically linear fashion. Therefore, for subsequent re-excision of 2 cm margin, not necessarily 2 cm has to be taken away from each tip of the longitudinal incisional scar. The surgeon needs to know the original size of the melanoma to reconstruct the melanoma within the context of the biopsy scar.

biopsies using a scalpel or skin punch. Further, it has been demonstrated that melanoma cells are not mechanically seeded into the dermis by punch biopsy using histochemical identification.[65] The main reasons to do an excisional biopsy are two fold: (1) although an incisional biopsy may establish the diagnosis of melanoma, a subsequent completion biopsy must be done in order to have the information on the thickness of melanoma; and (2) a small specimen will sometimes be difficult to make the diagnosis, especially true for acral lentiginous and lentigo malignant melanomas. For these reasons, shaved biopsy should be abandoned because shaving the entire level of the melanoma will compromise subsequent level and thickness determination. In general, if the lesion is smaller than 2 cm in diameter, it should be excised en toto with a 2 mm margin. However, if the lesion is larger than 2 cm or if it is at a site such as the face or digit that does not lend itself to excisional biopsy, an incisional biopsy using a scalpel or a skin punch is a reasonable approach. Patients with pigmented lesions often approach the dermatologist, who is frequently involved with the initial biopsy of a suspected mole. When the diagnosis is established, the patient will be referred to a surgeon for definitive surgical treatment. It is therefore important for a surgeon to interact closely with his dermatologist colleague so that the sequence of events can be traced to the time of biopsy. In this respect, the surgeon also works very intimately with his pathologist colleague to rely upon his judgment as to the thickness and level of the melanoma by which he recommends surgical treatment.

MULTIVARIANT MODEL

A multivariant model to predict the prognosis of melanoma has been established by Soong et al.[78] This model is based on a large data base of 4568 patients with stage I melanoma containing detailed clinical and pathologic information as well as long-term follow-up. Tumor thickness at diagnosis appears to be the single most important prognostic factor for the clinical outcome of these patients. Further, tumor ulceration, Clark's level, the anatomic site of the lesion and sex exert a significant influence on overall survival from diagnosis for some of the subgroups as characterized by tumor thickness. Tumor thickness at diagnosis is strongly indicative of melanoma recurrence and death, even following a disease-free interval of 2, 5 or 10 years. Anatomic site of the melanoma lesion and ulceration are of prognostic significance after disease-free intervals up to five years; however, their influence on melanoma recurrence and death is less significant after longer disease-free intervals.

INITIAL PATIENT EVALUATION

When a melanoma is diagnosed, the initial evaluation of the patient should include a complete history with emphasis in occupational or environmental exposure to sunlight as well as any accompanied conditions of immunological compromise. Further, a family history should be taken for about 10% of melanoma has a strong familial linkage.[48] This should be followed by a thorough physical examination, including a total body skin examination and palpation of the regional lymph nodes.

The emphasis of this evaluation is to identify risk factors, signs or symptoms of metastases, atypical moles and synchronous melanomas.

Initial workup consists of CBC, SMA20 and chest x-ray. For thin melanoma (<1 mm thickness), extensive diagnostic studies, such as computer axial tomography (CAT), magnetic resonance imaging (MRI) and nuclear scans, are not indicated. They are economically wasteful and should not be performed in staging these patients with thin primary melanoma.[60] However, for thicker melanoma or if there is suspicion that the patient has metastatic disease, appropriate scans should be undertaken.

The author has found MRI of the head and neck useful with a high-risk melanoma in the head and neck area, especially with clinically palpable cervical lymph nodes. The MRI may reveal additional deep-seated lymph nodes, which will be useful for surgical planning. Also, when axillary lymph nodes are palpated or if there is an equivocal finding of the axillary content, especially for obese patients, CAT scan of the chest with special attention to both axillas should be performed to evaluate the extent of nodal enlargement. In general, enlarged lymph nodes (over 1 cm) may be detected by CAT scans. If there is asymmetry of lymph node involvement, especially with the abnormal finding on the ipsilateral side to the primary melanoma, a lymph node dissection is indicated. When superficial inguinal lymph node is clinically suspicious, then abdominal and pelvic CAT scans should be performed to rule out deep inguinal lymph node involvement and intra-abdominal metastases.

SURGICAL TREATMENT OF STAGE I MELANOMA

It is important to know the Clark's level and particularly the Breslow's thickness of the lesion to guide the extent of re-excision. Further, it is imperative that the surgeon knows exactly the original size of the melanoma to reconstruct it within the context of the biopsy scar. The scar can be used as a reference point by which exact measurement can be derived to include it. Fig. 2 In general, the scar is thought to be potentially contaminated by microscopic tumor cells from previous biopsy, although, no conclusive data is available to demonstrate this. For this reason, a larger primary melanoma of greater than 2 cm should be biopsied with an incisional approach or a punch biopsy so that definitive surgery can be done with relatively smaller margin rather than having the field contaminated with a larger excisional scar. The rationale for wide excision of melanoma is based on the fact that complete removal of microscopic melanoma cells situated adjacent to the primary melanoma may result in decreased local recurrence and subsequent metastasis. Traditionally, a circumferential 5 cm margin from the tumor border was recommended. A report based on the World Health Organization's randomized study of 612 evaluable patients whose melanoma excisions showed that a 1 cm margin is safe for primary melanomas less than 1 mm thick in two groups randomized to 1 versus 3 cm margin.[17,77] However, the optimal margin for melanomas thicker than 1 mm has not been established. In the same WHO study, there were four local recurrences in patients whose melanomas were 1.0 – 2.0 mm thick with a 1 cm margin. On the other hand, the extent of excision, 1 cm versus 3 cm, showed no survival difference. For melanomas thicker than 2 mm, Aiken and associates[2] showed that survival was negatively effected if the excision margin was less than 2 cm. However, increasing the margin beyond 3 cm did not offer further advantage, and this finding was consistent with Ackerman's suggestion that occult metastases or microscopic satellitosis beyond 2 cm from the primary tumor may represent disseminated disease, and wider local excisions may not influence survival.[2] Further, high-risk primaries 1.7 mm or greater recur in 8–12% of patients even if the resectional margin is adequate.[69,82] After an adequate margin resection, additional margin is not statistically correlated with increased survival.[19,28,38,74] High-risk primaries have a risk for local as well as distant metastases. It appears that high-risk primaries have a high propensity of either lymphatic or hematogenous spread early, and therefore, even with adequate margin, the melanoma cells cannot be totally eradicated, and these cells as sites beyond the limit of the surgical margin will subsequently manifest as satellitosis or distant metastases. For practical purposes, it is important to define local recurrence in terms of persistent disease, which is defined as locally recurrent, usually in a scar and with a junctional melanocytic proliferation. It is biologically different from recurrent melanoma in dermis and also cutaneous fat, for example, as a microsatellite or intransit metastasis. Persistent disease is not, in general, a reflection of aggressive biological behavior, but rather inadequate surgical margins. On the other hand, recurrent disease may occur with adequate margins and reflects more aggressive biologic behavior. Microsatellites are sometimes found in sections of the primary site in tumors greater than 2.0 mm thickness. They appear to be more common than clinical satellitosis, but both

Table 1. Re-excision Margins for Primary Malignant Melanoma

Thickness	Margins (cm)*
Superficial Spreading or Nodular	
In Situ	0.5 - 1
≤ 1 mm	1
1 - 2 mm	2
≥ 2 mm	3
Lentigo Malignant Melanoma	
All	1

*Margins should be planned on complete biopsies of lesions. At anatomic sites where these rules cannot be applied, the widest practical excisional margin is reasonable.

situations are associated with a poorer prognosis.[25,28,38] Further, a local recurrence is associated with a high mortality rate of about 60–80%.[60] The melanoma intergroup lead by Balch et al has initiated a randomized clinical trial to determine whether 2 cm or 4 cm excision margins are appropriate for melanomas 1 mm to 4 mm thick. This study has been closed and is being evaluated. No published data is available at the time of publication of this book.[60]

Based on an extensive review of the literature, it has been accepted in most of the major melanoma centers that excision margins can be tailored to the thickness of melanoma and ulceration.[10,19,23,26,28,29,,30,53] The modified 1-2-3 rule, originally described by Fisher[29] as shown in Table 1 gives a general guideline for re-excision of melanoma with respect to thickness, so that 1 cm margin is allowed for thickness less than 1 mm; 2 cm margin for that between 1 and 2 mm; and 3 cm margin for that greater than 2 mm. It should be emphasized that margins should be planned only on complete biopsies of lesions and not on partial biopsies and recommendations should be modified to accommodate the anatomical sites and clinical circumstances. What might be appropriate for the back is usually not for the face. The above re-excision rule applies to superficial spreading and nodular types of melanoma. Other types such as lentigo malignant melanoma, desmoid plasty or acral lentiginous types may not be applicable.

Excision of the fascia is optional especially if it is convenient. Usually, with the exposed muscle, the wound can be closed easily, either primarily or with a skin graft. A retrospective study has been performed with melanomas of the trunk and proximal limbs in whom the fascia was removed in 107 and left intact in 95 patients by Kenady et al,[39] which showed no difference in survival. Since the lymphatics drain to the regional nodes through the subcutaneous tissue superficial to the deep fascia, removal of the fascia should not affect the incidence of recurrence or intransit disease. However, if it is used as a homogeneous deep margin for the excision, it would be easier to remove the fascia to ensure that all the fatty tissue would be removed. In certain cases, it would be technically difficult because the fascia is being incorporated in certain areas, such as in the origin of the muscle as the upper part of the tibialis anterior, the insertion of a muscle such as the iliotibial tract of the tensor fascia lata or the periosteum, such as in the anteromedial area of the tibia. Certainly when the primary melanoma is deeply invasive, the fascia should be removed. In fact, if it is a deep melanoma in the anteromedial area of the tibia, the periosteum may be removed as the deep margin.

Three approaches may be adopted to close the surgical defect: 1) a primary closure, 2) a split-thickness skin graft and 3) a full-thickness flap. In general, a wide excision of a melanoma in the shoulder or the anterior trunk or in the lateral chest wall can be encompassed by primary closure with elliptical incisional approach. However, in the upper extremities and in the lower extremities below the knee, sometimes it is difficult to close primarily, and therefore, skin graft may be performed. Fig. 2 shows sequential steps of a wide local excision of a previously melanoma-biopsied site using a split-thickness

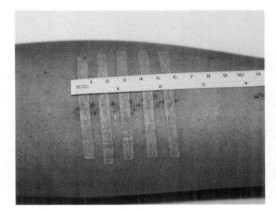

Fig. 2A.

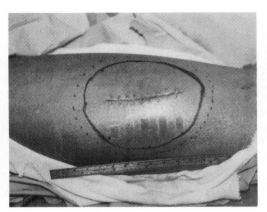

Fig. 2B.

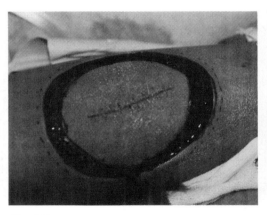

Fig. 2C.

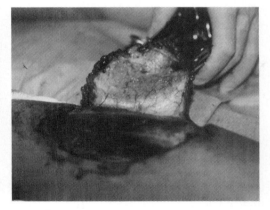

Fig. 2D.

Figs. 2A-J. This is a 17-year-old Caucasian female with a previously-biopsied nodular melanoma, Clark's level IV and Breslow thickness 2.5 mm in the left posterior calf. When the patient was referred to me, the longitudinal incision had healed well, measuring a total of 6 cm (Fig. 2A). The original mole measured 1 cm and was assumed to be in the center of the wound. It was decided that a 3 cm margin was needed to excise the melanoma biopsy site. Rather than taking 3 cm away from each point of the incisional scar, the center of the mole being assumed to be in the midpoint of the scar was the reference point to assume a 3 cm margin circumferentially. Therefore, the distance between the re-excision margin and each tip of the incisional scar was less than 3 cm since the biopsy had achieved additional distance in order to have an elliptical incision to be cosmetically closed (Fig. 2B). The dotted line shows the extension of subcutaneous tissue for an additional 1 cm of excision (Fig. 2C). Since there would be no significant consequence of taking the fascia, it was decided to remove the fascia as the deep margin (Figs. 2D-E).

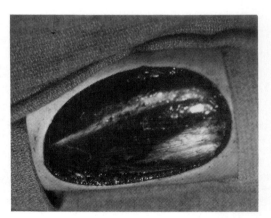

Fig. 2E.

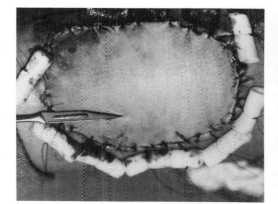

Fig. 2F.

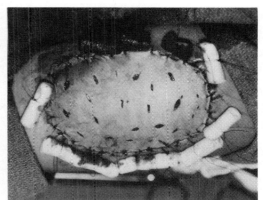

Fig. 2G.

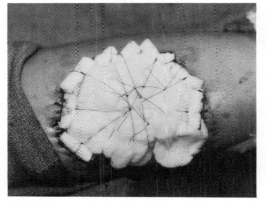

Fig. 2H.

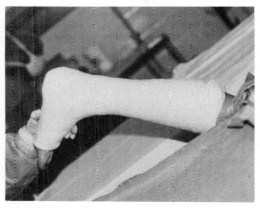

Fig. 2I.

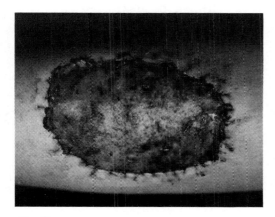

Fig. 2J.

A previously-prepared split-thickness skin graft was taken from the right upper lateral thigh using an air-driven Brown Dermatome of a thickness of 0.02 inch. This was used to cover the defect by interrupted sutures of 3-0 chromic sutures. The skin graft was punctured with a #11 scalpel to allow escape of blood or seroma (Figs. 2F-G). Alternatively, a 1:1 meshed split-thickness skin may be used. The skin graft was further bolstered by gauze soaked in mineral oil and secured with circumferential stitches of 3-0 nylon (Fig. 2H). A below-knee plaster cast was applied at the completion of the procedure to allow the patient to be discharged on postoperative day 1 without in-hospital immobilization (Fig. 2I). The patient returned to the clinic in 10 days, and the skin graft was noted to have a 100% take after the removal of the plaster cast (Fig. 2J).

skin graft. Even with skin graft, the patients can be discharged early by using plaster casting or splinting following local excision and skin graft.[47] For the seven patients studied the average hospital stay was 2.1 days rather than the usual 5–7 days of hospitalization for skin graft to take. This method has proved to be both financially beneficial and psychologically sound for patients with extremity melanoma requiring a wide local excision with skin graft. Because the surgical margins now are reduced with respect to the 1-2-3 rule, most surgical defects can be closed either by primary closure or reconstructive surgery using simple advancement flaps as well as more complex flaps, such as rotational flaps, rhomboid flaps and z-plasty.[43] In general, primary closure should be the goal in most anatomical sites as it is preferable for cosmetic and psychological reasons. A full-thickness flap closure gives better cosmetic results and padding over bony prominences or tendons as compared with a split-thickness skin graft.

In most instances, definitive re-excision of a primary melanoma can be achieved through outpatient surgery. The choice of local, regional or general anesthesia should be left to the individual judgment of the surgeon, anesthesiologist and the patient.

EXCISION OF MELANOMA AT SPECIAL SITES

Face. Because of the closeness to adjacent vital anatomic structures and cosmetic reasons, the margins used to excise facial melanomas are usually limited. Every attempt should be made to close the wound primarily. The other options would be rotational flaps and full-thickness skin graft. For lentigo malignant melanoma, which commonly occurs on the face, and fortunately has a low-risk of recurrence, usually a 1 cm margin of re-excision is adequate. For a large lentigo malignant melanoma, radiation therapy may be used as an alternative option to surgery.[34]

Ear. Melanoma of the ear can be excised by wedge re-excision or partial amputation of the ear.[16] Total amputation of the ear should be avoided, except for large recurrences or initially widespread disease. The most important consideration in the ear is to achieve an adequate re-excision. The upper part of the ear should be preserved as much as possible, especially for patients wearing glasses. An ear prosthesis may improve the cosmetic and psychological outcomes if indeed a total amputation of the ear is needed.[77]

Breast. To date, it has been established that primary melanoma of the breast should be treated as a local site like any other part of the body. Therefore, total mastectomy is not appropriate.[4,46,64,70] As at any other anatomical sites, the margins of re-excision of a breast melanoma should be planned on tumor thickness and removal of the entire breast is not appropriate.

Fingers and Toes. The principle of excising melanomas located on the fingers, especially on the thumb, is to remove as much of the digit as possible to achieve adequate margin and yet to preserve maximal function of the digit. If the melanoma occurs at the nail bed, the digit is preferentially amputated proximal to the distal interphalangeal joint with at least a 1 cm skin margin. In general, less skin is taken on the flexor surface so that a flexor or volar flap can be developed to close the skin. This approach is particularly helpful for the thumb so that the proximal phalanx can be preserved to retain significant function. When the melanoma is large and is not confined to the nailbed with more proximal extension or associated with satellitosis, metacarpophalangeal joint amputation (Ray amputation) is indicated. For melanoma on a toe either involving the nail or the rest of the digit, amputation of the entire digit at the metatarsophalangeal joint will provide the best local tumor control without significant functional loss.[58,62,63,77]

Sole of the Foot. Melanomas on the plantar surface of the foot of the acral lentiginous type often involve a large area; split-thickness skin grafts are oftentimes needed to close the excisional wound. It should be emphasized that the deep fascia over the extensor tendons should be preserved to support the skin graft. In this instance, the fascia should not be removed. If possible, especially if the tumor is relatively superficial and does not involve the deep fatty layer, a portion of the heel or ball of the foot should be retained for weight-bearing. If the primary surgery is done correctly, oftentimes muscle transposition flaps for heel coverage are not needed. It is rare to require amputation of the foot in order to excise primary melanoma of the foot.[58,77]

Penis. Distal penile cutaneous melanoma can be resected by a distal penectomy. Total penectomy should be avoided as much as possible.[72]

Mucosal Melanomas. Mucosal melanomas in the head and neck, the female genital tract (e.g. vulva and vaginal melanoma), the anorectum, the urethra and esophagus are relatively rare and account for about 3–4% of all melanomas diagnosed yearly[76] and require specialized approaches for the treatment of these sites. The characteristics of mucosal melanomas will not be covered in this chapter. The readers are referred to other sources[72] for in depth coverage.

IDENTIFICATION OF REGIONAL LYMPH NODES AT RISK

Extremity melanomas are relatively more predictable with respect to lymphatic drainage than the head and neck and trunk melanomas as upper and lower extremity would usually drain to the axilla and the inguinal area respectively. In general, head and neck melanomas often drain to the ipsilateral cervical lymph node chain. Melanomas on the anterior scalp, face and ear may have lymphatic drainage pathway to the parotid nodes as well. On the other hand, melanomas on the posterior scalp may drain to the occipital and retroauricular nodes in addition to the cervical lymph nodes. It should be noted that lymphatic drainage crossing the midline in the head and neck area is not uncommon. The same situation applies to trunk melanomas with possible drainage pathway to four major nodal basins, depending on the location of the primary melanoma. Sappey's line[73] gives a general guideline clinically to the direction of lymphatic drainage of melanoma in the trunk.[80] This is an imaginary line that runs from 2 cm above the umbilicus, curving slightly upward to the level of the second and third lumbar vertebra to form a band around the trunk. Both Sappey's line and the midline (Fig. 3) will divide the melanoma sites into four major quadrants with each quadrant draining to the corresponding regional lymph node. However, a minority of patients defy this rule in that their midline lesions may drain to all four nodal areas, especially those with primary sites in the umbilical area or midline back.[18] For this reason, a band of 4 cm in the midline and along Sappey's line (Fig. 3) may divide the nodal drainage areas more reliably. Further, a technetium-99 m antimony cutaneous scan may define the location of nodes that are the primary drainage of melanoma located anywhere on the trunk more accurately with injection of the radionuclide material at the primary melanoma site.[44,52] In general, an elective lymph node dissection for two nodal basins, as in both axillary nodal chain, requiring bilateral axillary dissection may be performed for trunk melanomas as detected by radionuclide scan. However, removing more than two nodal basins or bilateral neck dissection in an elective fashion is never indicated. Further, a bilateral inguinal dissection is usually not advised in an elective fashion because of its associated morbidity with edema of extremities and genitalia.

ELECTIVE LYMPH NODE DISSECTION FOR MELANOMA OF THE EXTREMITIES: PROS AND CONS

Even though the predicted regional lymph node involvement for upper and lower extremity melanoma is the axillary and the inguinal site respectively, the exact indication for elective lymph node dissection is still controversial, especially for the intermediary thickness group from 1.5 to 4 mm. However, over a large series

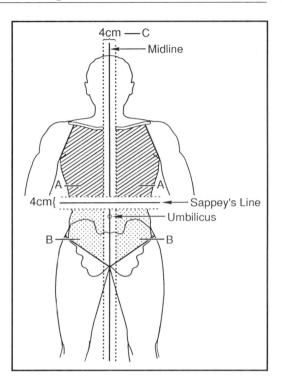

Fig. 3. Sappey's line and the midline divide the melanoma sites into four major quadrants with each quadrant draining to the corresponding regional lymph node. However, a minority of patients may defy this rule in that their midline lesions may drain to all four nodal areas, especially those with primary sites in the umbilical area or midline back (modified from Cascinelli, Vaglini, Nava, Santinami, Marolda).[18]

of studies, it has been shown that lymph node involvement with malignant melanoma less than 1 mm thick is quite rare, and therefore, elective lymph node dissection is not indicated in thin melanoma of less than 1 mm. On the other hand, thickness over 4 mm shows a significant increase in systemic involvement. Although the yield for microscopic lymph node involvement is high (62%) in this group, the rationale for not doing an elective dissection is that the overall survival will not be benefitted because of concomitant systemic involvement (72%).[7] Since controversy still exists with respect to extremity melanoma with a defined regional lymph node drainage pathway, other anatomical sites, including head and neck and trunk, with possible varied watershed lymphatic drainage patterns, make the data even more difficult to analyze in a retrospective fashion.

When the regional lymph nodes are palpated clinically to be enlarged consistent with melanoma, a dissection of the regional local lymph node chain is termed "therapeutic" or "delayed" lymph node dissection. On the other hand, when the regional lymph node examination is normal by clinical examination and yet potential risk of microscopic metastasis is present, an "elective" or "prophylactic" lymph node dissection is performed. This eliminates microscopic metastases with the argument that if the microscopic disease is found only at the sites of the regional lymph node, then extirpation of such microscopic disease may result in survival benefit.[9,11,12,53,66] Despite numerous publications,[8,21] the therapeutic benefits of elective lymph node dissection for clinical stage I melanoma are still controversial. Two large prospective randomized clinical trials are currently in progress,[7] which may provide additional valuable data regarding this controversy. However, the results of these studies will not be available for at least several years. A clear difference exists between the European practice and that of the United States, Australia and New Zealand. In Europe, a patient with melanoma is not likely to be offered an elective lymph node dissection, regardless of tumor thickness. On the other hand, in the United States, Australia and New Zealand, the majority

of patients, particularly those presenting to major melanoma centers, may be offered elective lymph node dissection if they have intermediate tumor thickness.[51] Patients with lentigo malignant melanoma are excluded because of their lower biological risk for metastases. According to Balch,[7] elective lymph node dissection should be reserved for selective patients with cutaneous melanoma of intermediate thickness (1.0–4.0 mm). This is especially true for 1.5–4.0 mm melanomas but more selectively for 1.0–1.5 mm lesions when elective lymph node dissection is confined to men with lesions on any anatomical site and women with trunk melanomas. However, others recommend that elective lymph node dissection is indicated for thick melanoma.[75] Since these conclusions are derived from retrospective studies, it is quickly pointed out by Balch[7,8] that a randomized prospective analysis for intermediate thickness melanomas of all anatomical sites addressed by cooperative cancer groups in the United States, Canada and Denmark would be important to provide unbiased data with respect to the role of elective lymph node dissection.

McCarthy et al[51] argue that it would seem reasonable to perform elective lymph node dissection for intermediate thickness tumors (>1.5 mm). In this group at least 56% will require lymph node dissection at a later date. For those in whom lymph node positivity is proven histologically, survival benefit would be considerably better than in those patients who have a delayed lymph node dissection for clinically positive nodes. Although it is true that 40% of patients may have unnecessary lymph node dissection,

McCarthy argues that this does not seem an unduly high price to pay when the benefits of dissection for clinically negative but histologically proved positive nodes are considered. A minimum benefit of 25% survival advantage can be expected for patients with intermediate thickness melanoma undergoing elective lymph node dissection. The authors further asserted that elective lymph node dissection is the treatment of choice for all melanoma patients with primary melanomas of greater than 1.5 mm in thickness until a large prospective randomized clinical trial which does not support elective lymph node dissection in this group of patients is published. On the other hand, Cascinelli et al argued against elective lymph node dissection[8,51] since the results have been conflicting with both opponents and proponents citing evidence to support each side of the issue.[22,31,33,50,55,59,79]

As these studies are not prospectively randomized clinical trials, there may well have been selection bias. The arguments against elective lymph node dissection may be summarized as follows.[51] 1) At least 70% of clinical stage I patients subjected to node dissection show no evidence of microscopic disease. 2) Systemic metastases do not always involve the regional lymph nodes. 3) It has never been proven that hematogenous spread arises from occult metastases in the regional lymph nodes. 4) Lymph node dissection may result in lymph edema which may favor the growth of residual tumor cells resulting in local recurrences or intransit metastases.

In an attempt to improve the percent detection of microscopic disease, Morton et al[57] devised a method using intraoperative identification of microscopic metastases in sentinel node (draining node nearest to the primary melanoma) by injecting marker dye to the primary melanoma site and removed by selective lymphadenectomy for intra–operative histologic diagnosis. They did not encounter true skin metastases in over 200 patients. In about 20% of the cases the sentinel node was positive and in about 80% of the cases it was negative. Therefore, they suggest that if the sentinel node is positive, complete en bloc lymph node dissection should be performed in an elective fashion. If the sentinel node is negative, the patient will be spared an extended operative procedure. Therefore, they argue that their method is reliable in dictating whether an operation should be done following identification of sentinel node, which is defined by the first echelon lymph node upon injection of dye in the local area of the primary tumor. However, this method is elaborate and requires a dedicated team of surgeons and pathologists. It is somewhat difficult apply widely in the treatment of melanoma.

CLINICAL SITUATIONS FOR ELECTIVE LYMPH NODE DISSECTION

Using predictive prognostic indications, if a patient is thought to benefit from by elective dissection, the selected patients should have minimal morbidity and virtually no mortality.[6,83] For elective lymph node dissection of the neck, either with or without the removal of the superficial parotid gland, a modified neck dissection is usually recommended.[14] A modified neck dissection spares the spinal accessory nerve, and therefore, the trapezius function should be preserved. Usually, the sternocleidomastoid muscle is preserved. However, the internal jugular vein is usually removed in a modified neck dissection. It is difficult to precisely predict the lymphatic drainage pathways to various parts of the neck as mentioned earlier. In general, a primary melanoma in the temporal or cheek area may drain into the preauricular, intraparotid, jugular digastric, midjugular, submandibular and submental lymph node chains. Therefore, neck dissection should include these nodal areas. A melanoma of the ear or the retroauricular area may drain into retroauricular, jugular digastric, jugular, posterior triangle and low jugular chain lymph nodes. A midoccipital melanoma may drain bilaterally to the retroauricular, suboccipital, subdigastric and posterior triangle. A bilateral posterior lateral neck dissection may be indicated in such a case. A unilateral occipital scalp melanoma may drain into the retroauricular, suboccipital posterior triangle and even anterior triangle lymph nodes. A chin melanoma may drain into the submental lymph node compartment, and therefore, a submental lymph node dissection may be indicated.[15]

When a melanoma is located in the arm or upper trunk, a standard radical axillary lymphadenectomy, including level I, II and III, should be performed.[3] The operative morbidity is extremely low (less than 5%).[8] For patients with melanoma of the leg or lower trunk, superficial lymph node dissection should be performed.[37] The iliac lymph node dissection should be avoided to minimize the problem of significant leg edema. However, if the superficial inguinal lymph nodes show multiple metastases, then an iliac lymph node dissection is indicated.

Using the above-described approach for lymph node dissection for different sites of melanoma, the overall operative morbidity is quite low and acceptable, especially in patients who will be benefitted by such a procedure.[24,33,36,83]

THERAPEUTIC LYMPH NODE DISSECTION

When regional lymph nodes are clinically positive for metastatic melanoma, a regional lymph node dissection will be considered therapeutic. If the metastatic workup is negative with a clinical stage II disease, then therapeutic lymph node dissection is indicated. Since surgery may achieve a 25–30% control rate for the disease and over 85% for regional nodal control, and there is no available systemic treatment to improve the statistics, an adequate lymph node dissection to extirpate the metastatic melanoma is crucial to achieve both excellent local control as well as potential long-term control for the patient. In general, the entire regional lymph node content should be removed en bloc along with the enlarged lymph node as a radical regional lymph node dissection, e.g. a radical neck dissection with ipsilateral involvement. Care should be taken not to enter the tumor, which could significantly increase the recurrence rate in the regional area. With multiple lymph nodes being involved and extracapsular involvement, postoperative adjuvant radiation therapy may be considered [Chapter 6].

FOLLOW-UP OF STAGE I MELANOMA PATIENTS

The prognosis for long-term survival for patients with early invasive melanoma (<1 mm) is excellent, over 95% for a 10-year period. Patients with recurrence tend to do so at local or regional sites that may still be amiable to surgical intervention. Overall, there is an increase of primary melanomas of about 3% in affected patients. The risk may be higher in patients with associated atypical moles and is particularly higher in affected members of melanoma-prone families (approximately 33%).[48] Therefore, these patients need a closer follow-up for the development of a second primary melanoma. Studies show that subsequent melanomas

diagnosed in a surveillance program are thinner than the incident melanoma.[49]

Follow-up of stage I patients consists of physical examination, including skin and lymph node sites, CBC and SMA20. Although no specific marker is available for melanoma, elevated serum lactate dehydrogenase (LDH) level is a useful marker of metastatic disease.[41] Clark's level may be used as a general guideline for the number of yearly follow-up visits.[56] Patients with high-risk melanoma or regional node metastasis should be seen at

---

Table 2. Clinical Stage I Melanoma Patients Follow-Up Based on Prognostic Risk Factors[20]*

1. *Low-Risk Primary*: Defined as >95% five-year survival

a.	Baseline Workup	Physical exam + CXR/CBC/SMA
b.	Examinations	q 6 months X 2 years, then annual (could vary with mole pattern)
c.	Laboratory	Repeat only prn

2. *Intermediate Risk Primary*: 75 – 95% five-year survival

a.	Baseline Workup	Physical exam + CXR/CBC/SMA
b.	Examinations	q 4 months X 2 years, q 6 months X 2 years, then annual
c.	Laboratory	Annual chest x-ray X 3 years Others repeat only prn

3. *High-Risk Primary*: Defined as <75% five-year survival

a.	Baseline Workup	Physical exam + CXR/CBC/SMA
b.	Examinations	q 3 months X 2 years q 4 months X 2 years q 6 months X 2 years, then annual
c.	Laboratory	CXR/CBC/SMA q 6 months X 3 years, then annual unless indicated CT or MRI if surgery (e.g. LND)** is indicated.

*These guidelines apply to superficial spreading and nodular melanoma. Other types are treated and followed differently, e.g. lentigo malignant melanoma, acral lentiginous and desmoplastic. Follow-up after recurrences must be individualized. **Lumph node dissection.*

Table 3. The Three-Stage System for Classification of Cutaneous Malignant Melanoma*

STAGE	ORIGINAL SYSTEM		MODIFIED SYSTEM
I	Localized primary melanoma		Local disease
Ia	Localized recurrence	Ia	Primary lesion alone
		Ib	Primary and satellites within a 5-cm radius of the primary
		Ic	Local recurrence within a 5-cm radius of the resected primary
		Id	Metastases more than 5 cm from primary but within the primary lymphatic drainage area
II	Regional nodal or in-transit metastases		Regional nodal disease
III	Disseminated disease		Disseminated disease

From Ketcham AS, Moffat FL, Balch CM. Classification and staging. In: Balch CM, Houghton AN, Milton GW, Sober AJ, Soong S-i, eds. Cutaneous Melanoma. Philadelphia: JB Lippincott, 1992; 213.

3–4 month intervals. Patients with atypical moles should be followed for second primary melanomas, and the baseline photographs for future comparisons may be useful.[60] Follow-up of atypical moles and serial photographs may be coordinated with a dermatologist who is interested in the management of early melanoma. Patients can assist in the management by performing self-examination of the skin on a monthly basis. In addition, patients with the diagnosis of melanoma should be encouraged to avoid excessive sun exposure and to use protective clothing and sunscreens, for example,

#15. Patients with atypical moles or positive family history should be enrolled along with their family members into a regular screening program, which may be supervised by a competent dermatologist. Despite the fact that the prognosis of thin melanoma (less than 1.0 mm in thickness), is excellent, there are a few that may recur over a long period of time.[68,84] Therefore, for melanoma including the thin group, they should be followed throughout the patient's lifetime. At the UCSF Melanoma Center, we adopt a follow-up scheme based on prognostic risk factors with respect to superficial

Table 4. The M.D. Anderson Cancer Center Staging System for Cutaneous Melanoma*

STAGE	CRITERIA	
I	Primary melanoma	
	IA:	Intact primary melanoma
	IB:	Primary melanoma, locally excised
	IC:	Multiple primaries
II	Local recurrence or local metastases within 3 cm of primary site	
III	Regional metastases	
	IIIA:	Tissues excluding nodes
	IIIB:	Node(s)
	IIIAB:	Skin etc. plus node(s)
IV	Distant metastases	
	IVA:	Cutaneous metastases only
	IVB:	Any visceral metastases

* *From Smith JL: Histopathology and biological behavior of melanoma. In Neoplasms of the Skin and Malignant Melanomas. Chicago, Year Book Medical Publishers, 1976.*

spreading and nodular melanoma. Based on clinical and microstaging data, three groups consisting of low, intermediate and high-risk primary may be divided.[20] They may be followed according to the scheme as shown in Table 2.

STAGING OF MELANOMA

One of the major barriers to a clearer understanding of cutaneous melanoma and its treatment is the lack of a comprehensive staging system which is universally accepted.[40] A melanoma staging system should include all manifestations of the disease with biologic predictive value, yet it must at the same time be simple enough to be adopted universally. It was in the

pursuit of this goal that prompted the American Joint Committee on Cancer (AJCC) and Union Internationale Contre le Cancer (UICC) to jointly propose a single pTNM (primary tumor, nodes and metastases) staging system for cutaneous melanoma. Traditionally, melanoma has been classified using the three-stage systems shown in Table 3. The MD Anderson Cancer Center Staging System for cutaneous melanoma has won popularity because of its simplicity and better delineation between stage III and stage IV disease (Table 4). However, these two staging systems do not take into account the Clark's levels and Breslow's thickness. Since microstaging is important in the prediction of melanoma, both the AJCC and UICC staging systems try to include the microstaging status in addition to the clinical status. In 1988 both the AJCC and UICC proposed the pTNM staging system for cutaneous melanoma as shown in Table 5. For a major melanoma center, it is recommended that a form (Fig. 4) as published by the American College of Surgeons and the AJCC for the new AJCC/ UICC pTNM 4-stage system should be followed. Although this system is more complicated than the traditional three-stage or M.D. Anderson staging system, it is currently the most comprehensive and the most updated format for staging malignant melanoma, both from a micro-staging and clinical point of view. Hope-fully, it is the starting point from which a universally accepted and utilized stag-ing system may evolve so that more mean-ingful data may be obtained in future clinical trials.

CONCLUSION

Microstaging of melanoma is the most reliable system to predict the prognosis of melanoma to date. Surgical treatment should be planned according to micro-staging data. Surgery remains the most effective treatment for primary melanoma, and for thin melanoma, surgery is cura-tive. Usually, a 1-2-3 rule is applied for the extent of excisional margin for

Table 5. The 1988 AJCC/UICC pTNM Staging System*

STAGE	CRITERIA
IA	Primary melanoma ≤0.75 mm thick and/or Clark's level II (pT1); no nodal or systemic metastases; N0, M0
IB	Primary melanoma 0.76 to 1.50 mm thick and/or Clark's level III (pT2); N0, M0
IIA	Primary melanoma 1.51 to 4.00 mm thick and/or Clark's level IV (pT3); N0, M0
IIB	Primary melanoma >4.0 mm thick and/or Clark's level V (pT4); N0, M0
III	Regional lymph node and/or in-transit metastases (any pT, N1 or N2, M0)
IV	Systemic metastases (any pT, any N, M1)

The AJCC Melanoma Committee recommends that when there is a discordance between thickness and level, the measured tumor thickness shall take precedence and be used for pT staging.

MELANOMA OF THE SKIN (EXCLUDING EYELID)

Data Form for Cancer Staging

Patient identification
Name _____
Address _____
Hospital or clinic number _____
Age _____ Sex _____ Race _____

Institution identification
Hospital or clinic _____
Address _____

Oncology Record

Anatomic site of cancer _____
Histologic type _____
Grade (G) _____
Date of classification _____

Chronology of classification
(use separate form for each time staged)
[ ] Clinical (use all data prior to first treatment)
[ ] Pathologic (if definitively resected specimen available)

Definitions

Primary Tumor (pT)

[ ] pTX   Primary tumor cannot be assessed
[ ] pT0   No evidence of primary tumor
[ ] pTis   Melanoma *in situ* (atypical melanotic hyperplasia, severe melanotic dysplasia), not an invasive lesion (Clark's Level I)
[ ] pT1   Tumor 0.75 mm or less in thickness and invades the papillary dermis (Clark's Level II)
[ ] pT2   Tumor more than 0.75 mm but not more than 1.5 mm in thickness and/or invades to papillary-reticular dermal interface (Clark's Level III)
[ ] pT3   Tumor more than 1.5 mm but not more than 4 mm in thickness and/or invades the reticular dermis (Clark's Level IV)
    [ ] pT3a   Tumor more than 1.5 mm but not more than 3 mm in thickness
    [ ] pT3b   Tumor more than 3 mm but not more than 4 mm in thickness
[ ] pT4   Tumor more than 4 mm in thickness and/or invades the subcutaneous tissue (Clark's Level V) and/or satellite(s) within 2 cm of the primary tumor
    [ ] pT4a   Tumor more than 4 mm in thickness and/or invades the subcutaneous tissue
    [ ] pT4b   Satellite(s) with 2 cm of primary tumor

Lymph Node (N)

[ ] NX   Regional lymph nodes cannot be assessed
[ ] N0   No regional lymph node metastasis
[ ] N1   Metastasis 3 cm or less in greatest dimension in any regional lymph node(s)
[ ] N2   Metastasis more than 3 cm in greatest dimension in any regional lymph node(s) and/or in-transit metastasis
    [ ] N2a   Metastasis more than 3 cm in greatest dimension in any regional lymph node(s)
    [ ] N2b   In-transit metastasis
    [ ] N2c   Both (N2a and N2b)

Distant Metastasis (M)

[ ] MX   Presence of distant metastasis cannot be assessed
[ ] M0   No distant metastasis
[ ] M1   Distant metastasis
    [ ] M1a   Metastasis in skin or subcutaneous tissue or lymph node(s) beyond the regional lymph nodes
    [ ] M1b   Visceral metastasis

Stage Grouping

[ ] I	pT1	N0	M0
	pT2	N0	M0
[ ] II	pT3	N0	M0
	pT4	N0	M0
[ ] III	Any pT	N1	M0
	Any pT	N2	M0
[ ] IV	Any pT	Any N	M1

Histopathologic Grade (G)

[ ] GX   Grade cannot be assessed
[ ] G1   Well differentiated
[ ] G2   Moderately well differentiated
[ ] G3   Poorly differentiated
[ ] G4   Undifferentiated

Histopathologic Type

The types of malignant melanoma are as follows:

Lentigo maligna (Hutchinson's freckle)
Radial spreading (superficial spreading)
Nodular
Acral lentiginous
Unclassified

    A rare desmoplastic variant also exists.
    Melanomas are identified according to site (mucosal, ocular, vaginal, anal, urethral, and so forth). The staging classification described in this chapter applies only to those arising in the skin.

Sites of Distant Metastasis

Pulmonary   PUL
Osseous   OSS
Hepatic   HEP
Brain   BRA
Lymph nodes LYM
Bone marrow MAR
Pleura   PLE
Peritoneum   PER
Skin   SKI
Other   OTH

Staged by _____ M.D.
_____ Referral
Date _____

Fig. 4. Reprinted with permission from Balch CM, Houghton AN, Milton GW, Sober AJ, Soong S-j, eds. Cutaneous Melanoma. Philadelphia: JB Lippincott, 1992:218. This is a standardized form published by the American College of Surgeons and the AJCC for the new AJCC/UICC pTNM4-stage system. The printing error made in stage grouping on the original form has been corrected in this reproduction.

melanoma with 1 mm, 2 mm and 3 mm of thickness to be resected with a 1 cm, 2 cm and 3 cm margin respectively. For thin melanoma less than 1 mm, no elective lymph node dissection is warranted. However, for melanoma with thickness greater than 1 mm, the role of elective lymph node dissection is controversial and should be individualized. All melanoma patients should be followed indefinitely for fear of late recurrence. In order to compare patients in well designed protocols a new staging system including micro-staging and clinical characteristics should be adopted as widely as possible.

REFERENCES

1. Ackerman AB, Scheiner AM. How wide and deep is wide and deep enough? Hum Pathol 1983; 14:743.

2. Aiken DR, Clausen K, Klein JP, James AG. The extent of primary melanoma excision: A reevaluation—how wide is wide? Ann Surg 1983; 198:634.

3. Ames FC, Balch, CM, McCarthy WH. Axillary lymph node dissection. In: Balch CM, Houghton AN, Milton GW, Sober AJ, Soong S-j eds. Cutaneous Melanoma. Philadelphia: JB Lippincott, 1992:384.

4. Ariel IM, Caron AS. Diagnosis and treatment of malignant melanoma arising from the skin of the female breast. Am J Surg 1972; 124:384

5. Bagley FH, Cady B, Lee A, Legg MA. Changes in clinical presentation and management of malignant melanoma. Cancer 1981; 47:2126.

6. Balch CM. Surgical management of regional lymph nodes in cutaneous melanoma. J Am Acad Dermatol 1980; 3:511.

7. Balch CM. The role of elective lymph node dissection in melanoma: Rationale, results, and controversies. J Clin Onc 1988; 6:163.

8. Balch CM, Milton GW, Cascinelli N, Sim FH. Elective lymph node dissection: Pros and cons. In: Balch CM, Houghton AN, Milton GW, Sober AJ, Soong S-j, eds. Cutaneous Melanoma. Philadelphia: JB Lippincott, 1992:345

9. Balch CM, Murad TM, Soong S-j et al. A multifactorial analysis of melanoma: Prognostic histopathological features comparing Clark's and Breslow's staging methods. Ann Surg 1978; 188:732.

10. Balch CM, Murad TM, Soong S-jet al. Tumor thickness as a guide to surgical management of clinical stage I melanoma patients. Cancer 1979; 43:883.

11. Balch CM, Soong S-j, Milton GW et al. A comparison of prognostic factors and surgical results in 1,786 patients with localized (stage I) melanoma treated in Alabama, USA, and New South Wales, Australia. Ann Surg 1982; 196:677.

12. Balch CM, Soong S-j, Murad TM,et al. A multifactorial analysis of melanoma: II. Prognostic factors in patients with stage I (localized) melanoma. Surgery 1979; 86:343.

13. Balch CM, Soong S-j, Shaw HM,et al. An analysis of prognostic factors in 8500 patients with cutaneous melanoma. In: Balch CM, Houghton AN, Milton GW, Sober AJ, Soong S-j, eds. Cutaneous Melanoma. Philadelphia: JB Lippincott, 1992:165

14. Byers RM. Cervical and parotid node dissections. In: Balch CM, Houghton AN, Milton GW, Sober AJ, Soong S-j, eds. Cutaneous Melanoma. Philadelphia: JB Lippincott, 1992:376.

15. Byers RM, Medina JE, Wolf PF. Regional node dissection of the head and neck. In: Balch CM, ed. Pigment Cell: Surgical Approaches to Cutaneous Melanoma. Switzerland: S Karger AG, 1985:83.

16. Byers RM, Smith JL, Russell N, Rosenberg V. Malignant melanoma of the external ear: Review of 102 cases. Am J Surg 1980; 140:518.

17. Cascinelli N, Adamus J, Balch C et al. Narrow excision (1 cm margin). A safe procedure for thin cutaneous melanoma. Results of an international randomized clinical trial. Arch Surg (in press).

18. Cascinelli N, Vaglini M, Nava M. Surgical treatment of melanoma of the trunk. In: Balch CM, ed. Pigment Cell: Surgical Approaches to Cutaneous Melanoma. Switzerland: S Karger AG, 1985:28.

19. Cascinelli N, Van der Esh EP, Breslow A et al. Stage I melanoma of the skin: The problem of resection margins. Eur J Cancer 1980; 16:1079.

20. Clark WH Jr, Elder DE, Guerry D IVet al. Model predicting survival in stage I melanoma based on tumor progression. JNCI 1989; 81:1893.

21. Cochran AJ, Wen D-R, Morton DL. Management of the regional lymph nodes in patients with cutaneous malignant melanoma. World J Surg 1992; 16:214.

22. Conrad FG. Treatment of malignant melanoma: Wide excision alone vs lymphadenectomy. Arch Surg 1972; 104:587.

23. Cosimi AB, Sober AJ, Mihm MC Jr, Fitzpatrick TB. Conservative surgical management of superficially invasive cutaneous melanoma. Cancer 1984; 53:1256.

24. Das Gupta TK. Results of treatment of 269 patients with primary cutaneous melanoma: A five-year prospective study. Ann Surg 1977; 186:201.

25. Day CL, Harrist TJ, Gorstein F et al. Malignant melanoma. Prognostic significance of "microscopic satellites" in the reticular dermis and subcutaneous fat. Ann Surg 1981; 194:108.

26. Day CL Jr, Mihm MC Jr, Sober AJ et al. Narrower margins for clinical stage I malignant melanoma. N Engl J Med 1982; 306:479.

27. Drzewiecki KT, Ladefoged C, Christensen HD. Biopsy and prognosis for cutaneous melanomas in clinical stage I. Scand J Plast Reconstr Surg 1980; 14:141.

28. Elder DE, Guerry D IV, Heiberger RM et al. Optimal resection margin for cutaneous malignant melanoma. Plast Reconstr Surg 1983; 71:66.

29. Fisher JC. Safe margins for melanoma excision. Ann Plastic Surg 1985; 14:158.

30. Goldman LI, Byrd R. Narrowing resection margins for patients with low risk melanoma. Am J Surg 1988; 155:242.

31. Goldsmith HS, Shah JP, Kim DH. Prognostic significance of lymph node dissection in the treatment of malignant melanoma. Cancer 1970; 26:606.

32. Grin-Jorgensen CM, Rigel DS, Friedman RJ. The worldwide incidence of malignant melanoma. In: Balch CM, Houghton AN, Milton GW, Sober AJ, Soong S-j, eds. Cutaneous Melanoma. Philadelphia: JB Lippincott, 1992:27.

33. Gumport SL, Harris MN. Results of regional lymph node dissection for m-

elanoma. Ann Surg 1974; 170:105.

34. Harwood AR. Conventional fractionated radiotherapy for 57 patients with lentigo maligna and lentigo maligna melanoma. Int J Radiat Oncol Biol Phys 1983; 9:1019.

35. Ho VC, Milton GW, Sober AJ. Biopsy of melanoma. In: Balch CM, Houghton AN, Milton GW, Sober AJ, Soong S-j, eds. Cutaneous Melanoma. Philadelphia: JB Lippincott, 1992:264.

36. Holmes EC, Moseley HS, Morton DL et al. A rational approach to the surgical management of melanoma. Ann Surg 1977; 186:481.

37. Karakousis CP Groin dissection. In: Balch CM, Houghton AN, Milton GW, Sober AJ, Soong S-j, eds. Cutaneous Melanoma.. Philadelphia: JB Lippincott, 1992:392.

38. Kelly JW, Sagebiel RW, Calderon W et al. The frequency of local recurrence and microsatellites as a guide to re-excision margins for cutaneous melanoma. Ann Surg 1984; 200:759.

39. Kenady DE, Brown BW, McBride CM. Excision of underlying fascia with a primary malignant melanoma. Surgery 1982; 92:615.

40. Ketcham AS, Moffat FL, Balch CM. Classification and staging. In: Balch CM, Houghton AN, Milton GW, Sober AJ, Soong S-j, eds. Cutaneous Melanoma. Philadelphia: JB Lippincott, 1992:213.

41. Khansur T, Sanders J, Das SK. Evaluation of staging workup in malignant melanoma. Arch Surg 1989; 124:847.

42. Kopf AW, Rigel DS, Friedman RJ. The rising incidence and mortality rate of malignant melanoma. J Dermatol Surg Oncol 1982; 8:760.

43. Kroll SS. Plastic surgical repairs of melanoma defects. In: Balch CM, Houghton AN, Milton GW, Sober AJ, Soong S-j, eds. Cutaneous Melanoma. Philadelphia: JB Lippincott, 1992:275.

44. Lamki LM, Logic JR. Defining lymphatic drainage patterns with cutaneous lymphoscintigraphy. In: Balch

CM, Houghton AN, Milton GW, Sober AJ, Soong S-j, eds. Cutaneous Melanoma. Philadelphia: JB Lippincott, 1992:367.

45. Lederman JS, Sober AJ. Does biopsy type influence survival in clinical stage I cutaneous melanoma? J Am Acad Dermatol 1985; 13:983.

46. Lee YN, Sparks FC, Morton DL. Primary melanoma of skin of the breast region. Ann Surg 1977; 185:17.

47. Leong SPL. Early discharge of patients following skin graft for extremity melanoma. J Dermatol Surg Oncol 1992; 18:204.

48. Lynch HT, Fusaro RM eds. Hereditary Malignant Melanoma, Boca Raton, FL: CRC Press, 1991.

49. Masri GD, Clark WH Jr, Guerry D IV et al. Screening and surveillance of patients at high risk for malignant melanoma result in detection of earlier disease. J Am Acad Dermatol 1990; 22:1042.

50. McCarthy JG, Haagensen CD, Herter FP. The role of groin dissection in the management of melanoma of the lower extremity. Ann Surg 1974; 179:156.

51. McCarthy WH, Shaw HM, Cascinelli N et al. Elective lymph node dissection for melanoma: Two perspectives. World J Surg 1992; 16:203.

52. Meyer CM, Lecklitner ML, Logic JR et al. Technetium-99m sulfur-colloid cutaneous lymphoscintigraphy in the management of truncal melanoma. Radiology 1979; 131:205.

53. Milton GW, Shaw HM, Farago GA, McCarthy WJ. Tumour thickness and the site and time of first recurrence in cutaneous malignant melanoma (stage I). Br J Surg 1980; 67:543.

54. Milton GW, Shaw HM, McCarthy WH et al. Prophylactic lymph node dissection in clinical stage I cutaneous malignant melanoma: Results of surgical treatment in 1319 patients. Br J Surg 1982; 69:108.

55. Moore GE, Gerner RE. Malignant melanoma. Surg Gynecol Obstet 1971; 132:427.

56. Morton D. Melanoma. In: Norton LW, Eiseman B, eds. Surgical Decision Making, 2nd ed. Philadelphia: WB Saunders Company, 1986:216.

57. Morton DL, Wen D-R, Wong JH et al. Management of clinical stage I melanoma by selective lymphadenectomy: Technical aspects. Arch Surg, in press.

58. Muchmore JH, Krementz ET, Reed RJ et al. Melanoma of the hand and foot (volar and subungual melanoma). In: Balch CM, Houghton AN, Milton GW, Sober AJ, Soong S-j, eds. Cutaneous Melanoma. Philadelphia: JB Lippincott, 1992:302.

59. Mundth ED, Guralnick EA, Raker JW. Malignant melanoma: A clinical study of 427 cases. Ann Surg 1965; 162:15.

60. NIH Consensus Development Conference. Diagnosis and Treatment of Early Melanoma, January 1992.

61. Nava M, Santinami M, Bajetta E et al. Melanoma cutaneo con metastasi ai linfonodi regionali (stadio II): Diagnosi, terapia, prognosi. Arg Onc 1982; 3:119.

62. Pack GT, Oropeza R. Subungual melanoma. Surg Gynecol Obstet 1967; 124:571.

63. Papachristou DN, Fortner JG. Melanoma arising under the nail. J Surg Oncol 1982; 21:219.

64. Papachristou DN, Kinne DW, Rosen PP. Cutaneous melanoma of the breast. Surgery 1979; 85:322.

65. Penneys NS. Excision of melanoma after initial biopsy. An immunohistochemical study. J Am Acad Dermatol 1985; 13:995.

66. Reintgen DS, Cox EB, McCarthy KS Jr et al. Efficacy of elective lymph node dissection in patients with intermediate thickness primary melanoma. Ann Surg 1983; 198:379.

67. Rigel DS, Kopf AW, Friedman RJ. The rate of malignant melanoma in the US: Are we making an impact? J Am Acad Dermatol 1987; 17:1050.

68. Ronan SG, Eng AM, Briele HA,. Thin malignant melanomas with regression and metastases. Arch Dermatol 1987; 123:1326.

69. Roses DF, Harris MN, Rigel D et al. Local and intransit metastases following definitive excision for primary cutaneous

malignant melanoma. Ann Surg 1983; 198:65-9.

70. Roses DF, Harris MN, Stern JS, Gumport SL. Cutaneous melanoma of the breast. Ann Surg 1979; 189:112.

71. Ross MI, Balch CM. General principles of regional lymphadenectomy. In: Balch CM, Houghton AN, Milton GW, Sober AJ, Soong S-j, eds. Cutaneous Melanoma. Philadelphia: JB Lippincott, 1992:339.

72. Ross MI, Stern SJ, Wanebo HJ. Mucosal melanomas. In: Balch CM, Houghton AN, Milton GW, Sober AJ, Soong S-j, eds. Cutaneous Melanoma. Philadelphia: JB Lippincott, 1992:325.

73. Sappey MPC. Anatomie, physiologie, pathologie des vaisseaux lymphatiques consideres chez l'homme et les vertebres. Paris: DeLahaye A, Lecrosnier. 1874.

74. Schmoeckel C, Bockelbrink A, Bockelbrink H et al. Low and high risk melanoma III. Prognostic significance of resection margin. Eur J Cancer Clin Oncol 1983; 19:245.

75. Schneebaum S, Briele HA, Walker MJ. Cutaneous thick melanoma. Arch Surg 1987; 122:707.

76. Scotto J, Fraumeni JF Jr, Lee JAH. Melanomas of the eye and other noncutaneous sites: Epidemiologic aspects. J Natl Cancer Inst 1976; 56:489.

77. Singletary SE, Balch CM, Urist MM et al. Surgical treatment of primary melanoma. In: Balch CM, Houghton AN, Milton GW, Sober AJ, Soong S-j, eds.

Cutaneous Melanoma. Philadelphia: JB Lippincott, 1992:269.

78. Soong S-j, Shaw HM, Balch CM et al. Predicting survival and recurrence in localized melanoma: A multivariate approach. World J Surg 1992; 16:191.

79. Southwick HW, Slaughter DP, Hinkamp JF, Johnson FE. The role of regional node dissection in the treatment of malignant melanoma. Arch Surg 1962; 85:63.

80. Sugarbaker EV, McBride CM. Melanoma of the trunk: The results of surgical excision and anatomic guidelines for predicting nodal metastasis. Surgery 1976; 80:22.

81. Urist MM, Balch CM. Head and neck melanoma. In: Balch CM, Houghton AN, Milton GW, Sober AJ, Soong S-j, eds. Cutaneous Melanoma. Philadelphia: JB Lippincott, 1992:295.

82. Urist MM, Balch CM, Soong SJ et al. The inference of surgical margins and prognostic factors predicting the risk of local recurrence in 3445 patients with primary cutaneous melanoma. Cancer 1985; 55:1398-1402.

83. Urist MM, Maddox WA, Kennedy JE, Balch CM. Patient risk factors and surgical morbidity after regional lymphadenectomy in 204 melanoma patients. Cancer 1983; 51:2152.

84. Woods JE, Soule EH, Creagan ET. Metastasis and death in patients with thin melanomas (less than 0.76 mm). Ann Surg 1983; 63.

CHAPTER 4

ISOLATED HYPERTHERMIC PERFUSION FOR MALIGNANT MELANOMA

Robert E. Allen, John C. Hutchinson,
Michele Pruitt Humel and Stanley P.L. Leong

For melanoma patients with local recurrence and intransit metastases of the extremities, isolated heated limb perfusion should be considered, especially where surgical resection could interfere with limb function. Isolated limb perfusion is also useful as adjuvant therapy in the treatment of high-risk acral lentiginous melanomas of the extremities.[1] This technique resulted from studies that infused nitrogen mustard into arteries supplying tumors while at the same time blocking the venous return to maximize exposure of the tumor to the chemotherapeutic agent.[2]

Further refined perfusion techniques were developed by Creech and associates.[3] A tourniquet was placed proximal to the point of perfusion and a heart-lung machine was added to circulate the perfusate and oxygenate the isolated extremity. By isolating the area, systemic toxicity was reduced and the response rate of the procedure was increased. This method allowed six to ten times the normal dose of drug that could be given locally to the cancer. The first report of a large series of patients treated with normothermic isolated perfusion with chemotherapy had survival of 20–25% better than patients who had been treated in the conventional way.[4]

A later development added heating to the isolated perfusion system, since heat can kill cancer cells, more than normal cells. The tumor killing effect of heat depends on the amount of heat and the length of time it is applied. Cavaliere and associates used heated blood perfusate in an attempt to improve the response rate from chemotherapeutic agents[5] They treated both sarcomas and melanomas, demonstrating an improved response rate. Since the reports of Cavaliere heat has been a part of the technique of isolated perfusion.

INDICATIONS FOR USE

The technique of isolated heated chemotherapy perfusion is applicable to cancers that are located in regions that can be isolated from the systemic circulation. In practice this usually means the arms and legs. Melanomas, sarcomas and some localized cutaneous lymphomas have been treated with this procedure. However, it has been applied most widely and effectively to cutaneous malignant melanoma.

Isolated heated limb perfusion is indicated in patients who present with extensive local tumors and certain high-risk primary lesions, such as acral lentiginous melanomas.[1] Locally recurrent melanomas, satellitosis, and in transit metastases are all grave prognoses and are best treated by perfusion.

TECHNIQUE OF ISOLATING THE LIMB

The principal advantage of isolated limb perfusion is the ability to deliver very large quantities of a cytotoxic agent to a localized tumor while sparing the rest of the body any significant drug toxicity. Melphalan (L-phenylalanine mustard) has been the most extensively used drug, either alone or in ion combination with other alkylating agents. Melphalan has many of the characteristics of an ideal agent for isolated limb perfusion. It is the least toxic of any other single agent. It has a short half-life, low toxicity to the vascular endothelium and soft tissues, limited cell cycle specificity, and a relatively linear dose response relationship for cytotoxicity.[6]

Prior to the induction of anesthesia and during anesthesia, the patients are warmed with an external heating devise (Blair Hugger) so that the patient's core temperature

is around 36°C. Preheating the patient shortens heating time during perfusion. The perfused extremity is wrapped in Saran Wrap during perfusion to decrease heat loss.

The technique begins with cannulating the arterial inflow and the venous outflow of the limb. For the upper extremity this means cannulating the axillary artery and vein, and in the lower extremity, the external iliac artery and vein. The femoral and popliteal vessels have been used also in the lower extremity. Isolation of the extremity is assured by the addition of a tourniquet around the root of the extremity. A 10 to 12 French AV cannula is used for the upper extremity perfusion and 12 to 18 French AV cannula for the lower extremity perfusions. The perfusion circuit consists of an Olson low flow modular pump, 1/4" I.D., 1/16" wall tygon arterial and venous tubing, a Bentley BOS-2S Oxygenator and an infant arterial line filter with filter bypass, a Heater-Cooler unit modified to heat to 50°C, and a Bentley model number therm-A arterial blood temperature probe. One hundred per cent oxygen and carbon dioxide is blended to achieve arterial PO_2 in the 300 to 500 mm Hg range and the PCO_2 in the 35 to 45 mm Hg range.

The extracorporeal circuit is primed with 500 cc of balanced electrolyte solution and the patient's own blood that remains in the isolated extremity. Three thousand units of beef lung heparin is added to the perfusate. The patient is heparinized systemically with 200 IU/kg of heparin. A rubber tourniquet is placed around the extremity and is held in place with a Galliger retractor (Fig. 1). Therefore, Stamin pins into the bony structures are not used. Needle thermistors are placed in the soft tissues at strategic locations to record the temperature of the extremity during the perfusion. Leakage of the perfusate into the general circulation is checked by injecting 2 ml of fluorescein into the perfusate and subsequent monitoring of leakage using a quantitative transcutaneous fluorescein monitor to access leakage intraoperatively.

The perfusate temperature is raised to 42°C and the temperature of the extremity is raised to 40°C and is not allowed to increase beyond those levels. Flow rates for the lower extremity are in the range of 400 to 600 cc/min and in the upper extremity of 250 to 350 cc/min (Fig. 2). Perfusion pressures should never be allowed to exceed systemic arterial mean pressures. Melphalan is added to the perfusate when the mean temperature near the tumor is 39°C. Perfusion is continued for one hour after the drug has been placed in the perfusate. Tourniquet time is limited to a maximum of two hours. The extracorporeal circuit is carefully monitored by a trained perfusionist. At the end of the perfusion the perfusate is drained

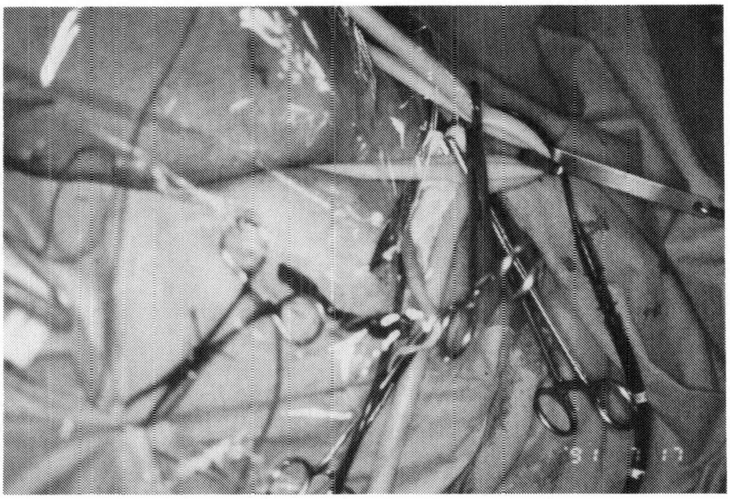

Fig. 1. Iliac perfusion and tourniquet in place. A rubber tourniquet is placed around the extremity and is held in place with a Galliger retractor.

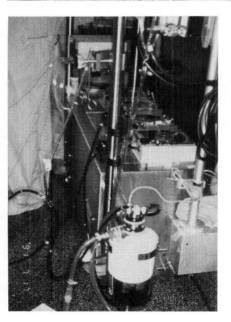

Fig. 2. Heart-lung machine for perfusion. The perfusion circuit consists of an Olson low flow modular pump, 1/4" I.D., 1/16" wall tygon arterial and venous tubing, a Bentley BOS-2S Oxygenator and an infant arterial line filter with filter bypass, a Heater-Cooler unit modified to heat to 50°C, and a Bentley model number therm-A arterial blood temperature probe.

and the extremity is washed out with a mixture of dextran 40 and balanced salt solution. The systemic heparin is reversed at the end of the procedure with protamine. Prophylactic fasciotimies are done at the end of the procedure.

Postoperatively the patient is kept at bedrest with the extremity elevated for three days and is treated with low dose heparin. Coumadin is started when the patient can eat orally to maintain a protime of 17 to 19 sec to minimize venous thrombosis. Oxygen saturation of the perfused extremity is continuously monitored for four days postoperatively. A fall in O_2 saturation usually means the start of a compartment syndrome and is an emergency since amputation may result if proper treatment is not prompt.

TECHNIQUE OF OPERATING PERFUSION PUMP

Satisfactory limb perfusion is almost exclusively dependent on the exact placement of the vascular cannulae, the venous being the more critical. The venous cannula must allow unencumbered flow from all the tributary veins of the limb, after placement of the tourniquet. Because the venous return conduit to the heart-lung machine is a fluid-filled descending tubing, there is a significant syphon-induced negative pressure in the venous cannula, which must not aspirate the vein wall in such a way as to kink off the venous outflow.

The arterial catheter must be as large as possible compared to the artery, so that its resistance does not raise the pressure excessively between the pump and the cannula. Line pressures in the order of 150 to 250 torr are common and safe, i.e., are well below pressures that could disrupt the arterial line.

After placement of the tourniquet, oxygenated warmed blood is pumped into the arterial cannula at a rate equal to the venous outflow, thus maintaining a steady reservoir volume. Flows of 10 cc per kilogram of body weight are common in femoral perfusions and about 5 cc per kilogram during axillary perfusions.

Inadequate venous drainage can be improved by elevating the foot 10 inches above the femoral vein. Repositioning of the venous cannula may be necessary if venous drainage remains unsatisfactory which leads to emptying of the oxygenator reservoir as arterial pumping rates are maintained. Lactated Ringer's solution can be added to the reservoir to compensate briefly for inadequacy of venous drainage; but this strategy will eventually lead to an excessive congestion of limb veins and foster a large volume of transudated fluid into the "third space."

It should be apparent that the perfusion rates are greatest in large limbs that are muscular and fat-free and smallest in older patients with small muscle mass and more fat per volume of limb. The flow in the leg may range from 400 to 2000 cc/min and in the arm from 100–400 cc/min. Monitoring the dorsalis pedis or radial artery pressure helps assess the adequacy of the flow. These distal arterial pressures generally remain well below the centrally measured mean arterial pressure; and this difference helps guarantee that if there is imperfect isolation of the limb by the tourniquet collateral blood transfer will tend to be toward the limb, rather than toward the systemic circulation, thus keeping the chemotherapy isolated.

Occasionally there is gradual accumulation of blood in the reservoir, indicating a venous return greater than the arterial pumping rate. The arterial pumping rate can be increased to compensate, watching that the line pressure does not become excessive or that the distal arterial pressure in the limb does not exceed the systemic mean arterial pressure. If the arterial flow seems maximal, the venous flow can be impeded by a screw-clamp resistor placed in the venous syphon line, while monitoring the resulting back pressure with a stand-pipe manometer. This venous line resistor will cause limb venous distension and could result in venous collateral flow past the tourniquet to the body, if excessive.

Isolation of the blood volume in the perfused limb from the central blood volume is judged by several observations. The first is stability of the oxygenator reservoir, indicating that perfusion is proceeding without the transfer of volume to the limb (and thus possibly to the patient), and without transfer of fluid from the limb (and thus possibly from the patients). Fluorescein, 5 ml, added to the perfusate, should not appear in the urine or tears when there is complete isolation of the limb. Fluorescein will be evenly distributed within the skin of the limb when the distribution of perfusion is even throughout the limb. This observation requires viewing the limb under ultraviolet light with the OR lights off.

Warming of the limb is achieved by heating the arterial blood to 42°C maximally. The arterial blood temperature thermistor must be calibrated against an accurate reference thermometer in order to prevent excessive blood heating. When tissue temperatures reach 39°–40°C, the chemotherapeutic agent, usually Melphalan, is added to the perfusate; and the perfusion is continued for one hour, while constantly monitoring tissue and blood temperature. Tissue temperatures in excess of 40°C lead to progressive vascular, neural and skin injury and to third space edema.

At the end of the recirculation period, the venous return is disconnected from the oxygenator and directed to a container for discard. The arterial inflow is continued while small (100–200 cc) additions to the oxygenator are made from a mixture of 500 cc Lactated Ringers and 500 cc of Dextran 40, thus "rinsing" the limb of the perfusate containing residual Melphalan. This procedure results in a venous effluent with a very low hematocrit. The amount of red cell loss to the patient can be estimated by the volume and hematocrit of the discarded perfusate. This loss can be replaced by transfusion to the central circulation if indicated.

Oxygenation of the perfusate is done using a gas mixture of about 20:1, oxygen to carbon dioxide. This results in hypercapnia of the perfusate with PCO_2's of 50 to 70, a range which causes a respiratory acidosis favoring vasodilation.

RESULTS OF TREATMENT

One hundred ninety-eight patients with melanoma of the extremities have been treated with isolated heated perfusion at UCSF from 1978 to 1992. The 5-year cure rate for patients with intransit metastases and negative nodes is 62%. The 5-year cure rate for acral lentiginous lesions is 75%, based on 61 patients being perfused. Patients treated by surgery alone without perfusion did much worse, as shown in Table 1,

Table 1. Personal data from the University of California, San Francisco. Patients treated by surgery alone without perfusion, 1972-1982

SURVIVAL: Local Recurrence Without Perfusion

°   Within 5 cm of primary
-    65 total patients
-    43 patients (66%) died within 5 years
-    22 patients (34%) survived 5 years or longer

°   Satellites
-    12 total patients
-    2 patients (17%) alive after 5 years

°   Intransit Metastasis
-    23 total patients
-    6 patients (26%) survived 5 years after diagnosis

from our data as well as from others.[7,8]

There is controversy regarding whether patients with high-risk stage I melanoma should have prophylactic perfusion or just surgery alone. There is one prospective randomized series which reports increased disease-free survival for stage I patients treated with perfusion.[9,10]

Perfusion, on the average, offers 20 to 25% increased survival over other modalities of therapy in patients who have stage II and III melanoma. Some reported ranges of survival after perfusion are shown in Table 2.[11,12]

COMPLICATIONS

About 30% of patients undergoing perfusion will experience complications. Most of the complications are minor and transitory. Severe hemopoietic toxicity occurs in approximately 5% of patients. This complication is usually temporary. Mortality from the procedure is low. Severe swelling of the extremity until there is compromise of the circulation (compartment syndrome) occurs in 3 to 4% of patients, and if the condition is not treated promptly, amputation will result. Edema occurs universally but if properly treated is not long-lasting. There is a high risk of postoperative hemorrhage since anticoagulation is used. Thrombophlebitis occurs in 15% of patients but pulmonary embolism is rare.

CONCLUSION

Isolated heated regional perfusion with chemotherapeutic agents is the treatment of choice for the very high-risk melanoma, locally recurrent melanoma and intransit metastatic melanoma. Its role in the very high-risk melanoma remains to be determined. Heat alters tumor cell membrane permeability, which in turn enhances intracellular drug uptake. There is a 2 to 3

Table 2. Five-year survival rate of extremity melanoma patients with different stages according to M.D. Anderson classification following perfusion.

STAGE	5-YEAR SURVIVAL
I	89 – 94 %
II	74 – 77 %
IIIA	70 – 81 %
IIIB	48 – 54 %
IIIAB	30 – 45 %
IV	20 – 25 %

log kill of tumor cells at 42°C over that at 37°C for several drugs, including thiotepa, phlenylalamine mustard, adriamycin and methyl-CCNU. Thus, there is synergism of hyperthermia and drug therapy.

This procedure is high-risk; however, when properly indicated, the benefits far outweigh the risks, and the majority of patients survive the procedure with increased long-term survival.

REFERENCES

1. Fletcher JR, White CR Jr, Fletcher WS. Improved survival rates of patients with acral lentiginous melanoma treated with hyperthermic isolated perfusion, wide excision, and regional lymphadenectomy. Am J Surg 1986; 151:593.

2. Klopp CG, Alford TC, Bateman J et al. Fractionated intra-arterial cancer chemotherapy with methyl bis amine hydrochloride: a preliminary report. Ann Surg 1950; 132:811.

3. Creech O Jr, Krementz ET et al. Chemotherapy of cancer: regional perfusion utilizing an extracorporeal circuit. Ann Surg 1958; 148: 616.

4. Stehlin JS, Clark RI Jr et al. Regional chemotherapy for cancer: Experiences with 116 perfusions. Ann Surg 1960; 151: 605-19.

5. Cavaliere R, Giocatto EC, Grovanella BC et al. Selective heat sensitivity of cancer cells: biochemical and clinical studies. Cancer 1967; 20: 1351.

6. Minor D, Allen RE et al. Pharmakinetics of isolated limb perfusion with heat and melphalan for melanoma. Am Soc Oncol 1983; 2: 239.

7. Stehlin JS Jr. Melanoma—Yesterday, today, and tomorrow: A 30-year perspective. Houston Med J 1988; 4:49.

8. Stehlin JS Jr, Greeff PJ, de Ipolyi PD et al. Heat as an adjuvant in the treatment of advanced melanoma: An immune stimulant? Houston Med J 1988; 4:61.

9. Ghussen F, Kruger I, Groth W, Stutzer H. The role of regional hyperthermic cytostatic perfusion in the treatment of the extremity melanoma. Cancer 1988; 61:654.

10. Koops, HS, Kroon BBR, Oldhoff J et al. Controversies concerning adjuvant regional perfusion for stage I melanoma of the extremities. World J Surg 1992; 16:241.

11. Krementz ET. Regional perfusion. Current sophistication: What next? Cancer 1986; 57:416.

12. Lienard D, Lejeune FJ. In transit metastases of melanoma treated by high dose of rTNF in combination with interferon— and melphalan in isolation perfusion. World J Surg 1992; 16:234.

CHAPTER 5

SURGICAL MANAGEMENT OF METASTATIC MELANOMA

Robert E. Allen, Jr.
and Stephen J. Mathes

Surgery is most effective when melanomas are localized. When melanomas become disseminated, the role of surgery is limited but very important in offering significant quick palliation that may at times result in prolonged survival. Melanoma metastases should be surgically removed when relatively simple resections can leave the patient clinically free of disease. Subcutaneous nodules should be resected when these lesions are enlarging and located in areas of the body, such as the face and extremities.

Some patients present with massive local cutaneous and subcutaneous melanoma that cannot be managed by the usual surgical approaches and cannot be contained by irradiation alone. Typically, these patients have minimal metastases elsewhere and are expected to live an extended period of time. Radical local excision of these tumors with closure of the defects with normal skin and muscle with its own blood supply is an effective way to manage this difficult situation. (Fig. 1) The areas of metastases as well as adjacent sensitized skin is replaced with normal skin.

LOCALLY RECURRENT MELANOMA

Traditionally, local recurrence of melanoma is considered to be the appearance of melanoma foci within 5 cm of the primary excision site. This includes metastatic melanoma involving the primary excision site, satellites and intransit metastases. It is important to distinguish local recurrence from local persistence of melanoma, which is considered to occur when the primary lesion was not adequately excised, the usual basis for litigation under the heading of "failure to diagnose". Survival following local recurrence is generally poor and often is the first warning of disseminated spread. Approximately two-thirds of patients with locally recurrent

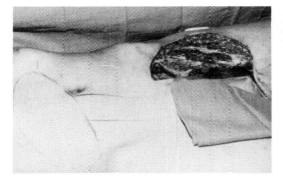

Fig. 1A

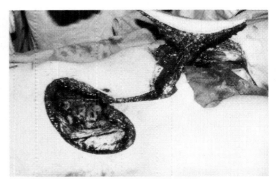

Fig. 1B

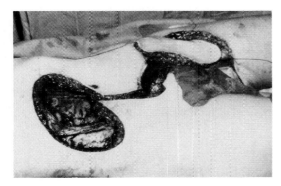

Fig. 1C

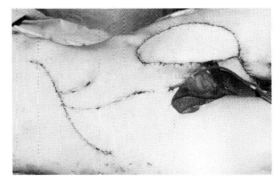

Fig. 1D

Fig. 1. Patient with invasive localized metastasis in groin. This was resected, and the defect was covered with a rectus myocutaneous flap.

melanoma can be expected to die from disseminated melanoma and of those with intransit melanoma spread, 80% will die from disseminated disease.[1,2]

The treatment options are: 1) surgical excision; 2) surgical excision with radiation; 3) radiation alone; and 4) isolated heated limb perfusion with regional chemotherapy. The treatment of choice for a single first local recurrence is surgical excision, particularly in a patient with previous low-risk primary or after a prolonged interval with no evidence of disease (NED). Additional radiation therapy may be indicated in areas where several satellites have appeared simultaneously or sequentially. This is often seen on the scalp and face and in areas where micro-scopic tumor is suspected to be present even after a wide excision.

Isolated heated limb perfusion is the treatment of choice for locally recurrent melanoma and for high-risk acral lentiginous melanomas of the extremities. A prospective study, although incomplete, has detailed the benefits of this procedure.[3] From our experience at the University of California, San Francisco, 5-year survival for locally recurrent, intransit and acral lentiginous melanoma patients is in the range of 60–65%, and the 10-year survival approaches 30–50%. It should be emphasized that this is a highly technical procedure that can only be done in a few tertiary care centers, and it is important for the dermatologic surgeon to know where the centers are and to be in touch with the directors when the possible need for this treatment modality comes up. A more detailed account of isolated heated limb perfusion has been described in chapter 4.

Laproscopic surgery is a new technique which is useful in examining the peritoneal and thoracic cavities when the CT scan is confusing or indeterminate. Biopsies of the liver and visual examination can be done. Laproscopic retroperitoneal lymph node biopsies and resection for staging are easily done with minimal morbidity and without hospitalization.

LYMPHADENECTOMY

Therapeutic lymph node dissection is not controversial. This procedure should be applied when there is clinical or pathological evidence that the regional nodes are involved. However, widespread metastases may militate against therapeutic lymphadenectomy.

Elective lymphadenectomy is a more complicated issue. Since the first place to which melanomas tend to spread are the regional lymph nodes, most patients with intermediate and high-risk melanomas (>1.5 mm) agree to have a regional lymph node dissection, especially in view of the slight associated morbidity (about 5%). Many surgeons and physicians espouse this position as a means to give the patient a survival advantage, and at the very least, to stage the disease and further hone prognosis factors. The majority of retrospective studies suggest that elective lymphadenectomy increases survival, but the results are not statistically significant. Our own unpublished data, expressly using

paired comparison outcomes, suggest 6–8% 5-year survival advantage for patients who received lymph node dissection vs those who did not. Two prospective non-randomized studies by the WHO and the Mayo Clinic reported no increased survival for patients who had elective lymph node dissections.[4,5] These studies, unfortunately, were flawed and cannot be accepted as the paradigm for lymph node dissection. The issues of this emotional debate are well-delineated in the second edition of *Cutaneous Melanoma*, edited by Balch et al.[6] Two new prospective randomized surgical trials have been conducted in North American and Europe, but the findings have not yet been reported. Until the results of these trials are published and scrutinized, elective lymph node dissection should be available for patients in the high-risk groups where there is a likelihood of minimal or microscopic melanoma metastases. Tumor thickness (2.5 mm to 4.5 mm), histologic grade, mitoses and location should be included in the decision process. The arbitrary cut-off point of 4 mm thickness by Balch et al for not doing elective node dissection due to the low-risk benefit ration[6] is not universally accepted. The 5-year survival of very high-risk patients at UCSF is 50%, so that aggressive therapy may improve this survival.

Once the decision is made to do a regional lymphadenectomy, there are options as to the extent of surgery. Axillary lymphadenectomy should involve all levels, including the highest axillary lymph nodes. Morbidity from this operation is low with incidence of arm edema less than 1%. Neck dissections should be functional and designed to remove the draining lymph nodes and spare normal structures usually sacrificed for technical reasons and ease of operation. These structures should only be sacrificed for completeness of the surgical operation. The operation should be as regional as possible, i.e. for a primary melanoma in the temporal area, the operation should include the superficial parotid gland as well as the lymph nodes of the upper neck. Usually it is not necessary to do a full neck operation.

Superficial groin dissection is preferred and is most commonly done. Radical groin dissection is not advised because the risk benefit ratio does not support the additional surgery. The morbidity of radical groin dissection is considerable and when the pelvic nodes are involved the 5-year survival is around 12%; therefore, elective pelvic node dissection is not justified. Recent reports indicate that as many as 30% of the lymph nodes reported to be negative for occult metastases may in fact be positive when careful techniques and special stains are used to study the specimen.[7] Recently, Morton and associates have reported a technique of injecting a vital blue dye intradermally at the primary site to accurately identify the "sentinel" node or group of nodes draining the primary basin.[8] These nodes are removed and subjected to frozen section. If they are positive, a lymph node dissection is done. This method may prove enormously beneficial because it could, if validated, sort out patients requiring lymphadenectomy from those without occult metastases.

The technique of minimal skin flap dissection in superficial groin dissections decreases the morbidity of skin necrosis and infection. (Fig. 2) The two incision techniques for radical groin dissection also

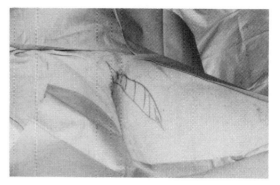

Fig. 2A

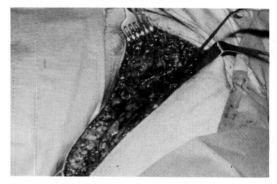

Fig. 2B

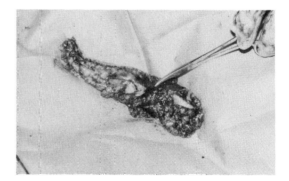
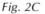

Fig. 2C

Fig. 2A-C. Superficial groin dissection technique of minimal flap development. An elliptical incision was made to include the central strip of skin of the femoral triangle. (Fig. 2A) Minimal flap was developed to the medial border of the sartorius and lateral border of the adductor longus. Dissection of the femoral triangle was carried out. (Fig. 2B) The specimen with the overlying skin is shown. (Fig. 2C)

significantly decrease leg edema. Edema of the leg should be anticipated and steps taken to prevent permanent edema immediately postoperatively by providing elevation and elastic compression.

RESECTION OF METASTATIC MELANOMA

The lung is frequently the site of melanoma spread and when these lesions are solitary, surgical intervention may be the treatment of choice since surgery is the only modality that offers prolonged palliation and a chance for cure. The median survival for lung metastases after surgery is 12 months and 5-years survival approaches 20%.[9]

Brain metastases occur late in the course of melanoma, and the majority of deaths from melanoma are attributable to brain involvement. Survival after brain metastases is measured in months. Some long-term palliation and survival can be obtained with surgical resection followed by irradiation to the whole brain. Recent advances in stereotaxic irradiation with precise delivery of x-rays through multiple ports may increase survival and palliation in this area.[10,11,12,13]

Metastases to the gastrointestinal tract are rarely solitary and are occult until hemorrhage or intestinal obstruction alerts the patient and physician. Here again, the palliative role of surgery offers a quick and effective method of treating these emergencies.[14]

Treatment decisions in the disseminated phase of metastatic melanoma are best done with team input, weighing the options based on cost/benefit and quality of life. Sometimes the best therapy is no treatment. This is notably true in the very elderly or infirm patients or when the tumor is widely disseminated and moving rapidly. In some asymptomatic patients, this decision is made in order to maintain quality of life for as long as possible, when the outlook is particularly bleak for any realistic survival time. On the other hand, the decision to surgically debulk a lesion is occasionally made in order to allow other systemic therapies an opportunity to have an impact.

Table 1 contains data on the median and 5-year survival of lesions surgically removed from different sites.[15,16] The point to make is that cancer surgeons are becoming more aggressive in dealing surgically with distant metastases and have

TABLE 1. Prognosis After Surgery of Widespread Metastatic Melanoma

	MEDIAN SURVIVAL	5-YEAR SURVIVAL
Subcutaneous Nodules	19 months	25%
Lung	12 months	21%
Brain	6 months	20%
Intestine	11 months	22%
Solitary Metastases	24 months	30%
Multiple Metastases	7 months	8%

obtained some gratifying results in what previously had been considered a hopeless situation.

CONCLUSION

Surgery is the treatment of choice for most local recurrences. In widely disseminated diseases, surgery is still the option of choice, where feasible, and where it does not compromise the patient's quality of life in the last months of their life.

Other treatment modalities pale in effectiveness by comparison, and many new experimental approaches, such as the use of biological response modifiers and vaccines, are under trial to help correct the balance between medical and surgical care of advanced melanoma.

REFERENCES

1. Roses DF, Karp NS, Oratz R et al: Survival with regional and distant metastases from cutaneous melanoma. Surg, Gyn and Obs 1991; 172:262.
2. Markowitz JS, Cosimi LA, Carey RW et al: Diagnosis after initial recurrence of cutaneous melanoma. Arch Surg 1991; 126:703.
3. Ghussen F, Kruger I, Groth W, Stutzer H. The role of regional hyperthermic cytostatic perfusion in the treatment of the extremity melanoma. Cancer 1988; 61:654.
4. Versonesi U, Adamur J, Bandiera DC et al. Delayed regional lymph node dissection in stage I melanoma of the skin of the lower extremities. Cancer 1982; 49:2420.
5. Sim FH, Taylor WF, Pritchard DJ et al: Lymphadenectomy in the management of stage I malignant melanoma: A prospective randomized study. May Clin Proc 1986; 61:697.
6. Balch CM, Houghton AN, Milton GW et al, eds. Cutaneous Melanoma, 2nd ed. Philadelphia: JB Lippincott; 1992:345-66.
7. Heller R, Becker J, Wasselle J et al: Detection of submicroscopic lymph node metastases in patients with melanoma. Arch Surg 1991; 126:1455.
8. Cochran AJ, Weng D-R, Morton DL. Management of the regional lymph nodes in patients with cutaneous malignant melanoma. World J Surg 1992; 16:211.
9. Wong JH, Euhus DM, Morton DL. Surgical resection for metastatic melanoma to the lung. Arch Surg 1988; 123:1091.
10. Brega K, Robinson WA, Winston K et al: Surgical treatment of brain metastases in malignant melanoma. Cancer 1990; 66:2105.
11. Winston KR, Lutz W. Linear accelerator as a neurosurgical tool for stereotactic radiosurgery. Neurosurg 1988; 22:454.
12. Phillips MH, Frankel KA, Lyman JT et al: Comparison of different radiation types and irradiation geometries in stereotactic radiosurgery. Int J Rad Oncol Biol Phys 1990; 18:211.
13. Davey P, O'Brien P. Disposition of cerebral metastases from malignant melanoma: Implications for radiosurgery. Neurosurg 1991; 28:8.
14. Klaase JM, Kroon BB. Surgery for melanoma metastatic to the gastrointestinal tract. Br J Surg 1990; 77:60.
15. Branum GD, Epstein RE, Leight GS et al: The role of resection in the management of melanoma metastatic to the adrenal gland. Surgery 1991; 109:127.
16. Cauty GC, Donohue JH, Goellner JR et al: Metastatic melanoma of the gastrointestinal tract. Arch Surg 1991; 126:1353.

CHAPTER 6

RADIATION THERAPY FOR MELANOMA

Patrick S. Swift
and Karen K. Fu

The effective integration of radiation therapy into the overall approach to malignant melanoma has long been hampered by the belief that melanoma is a radioresistant tumor. Such a belief is indefensible in light of clinical information garnered over the past two decades. In a recent Radiation Therapy Oncology Group (RTOG) trial, randomizing patients with measurable metastatic melanoma lesions to two different radiation fractionation schemes, complete responses were seen in 24% of cases, and partial responses in an additional 35%.[59] Prior retrospective studies have reported complete response rates of 22–47%,[28,36,42,49,67] with an 80–87% chance of retaining control at five years.[42,49] Evidence such as this clearly indicates that some melanomas respond well to radiation. The difficulty lies in the fact that not all melanomas respond in a similar fashion to radiation therapy due to radiobiological variations between individual tumor cell lines.

THE RADIORESPONSIVENESS OF MELANOMA

Initial attempts to explain the lack of a clear cut responsiveness to radiotherapeutic intervention built upon the radiation cell survival curves established for four different melanoma cell lines from Dewey and Baranco.[5,15] All four cell lines were found to have radiation cell survival curves characterized by a large extrapolation number, n (25–40), and a low mean lethal dose, D_0 (85–100), with a broader shoulder than had previously been seen for other tumors studied. (Table 1) This suggested an increased capacity for repair of sublethal damage between fractions of radiation, leading clinical radiation oncologists to arrive at the conclusion that larger fraction sizes might be necessary to improve response. In the ensuing years, several

Table 1. Survival Curve Parameters of Human Melanoma Cells Irradiated in Vitro[56]

D_o	0.62 – 2.11 Gy
D_q	0 – 3.69 Gy
n	1 – 40
α	0 – 0.88 (Gy^{-1})
β	0.008 – 0.180 $(GY^{-2}$
α / β	0.6 – 63.8 Gy

retrospective analyses were carried out which strongly suggested an advantage to the use of larger individual fraction sizes (4–8 Gy) over conventional daily doses (1.8–2.5 Gy).[28,36,49,51]

In Overgaard's review of 204 lesions in 114 patients,[51] only 24% of patients treated with individual fraction sizes less than 4 Gy were complete responders, compared with 57% complete responders among those treated with fraction sizes ≥ 4 Gy . Duration of treatment and total dose did not appear to influence response rates. Dose per fraction and tumor volume were the strongest predictors of response. In 45 of these patients, who had all known disease encompassed in the local radiation fields, a three-year survival rate of 31% was noted with an overall local control rate of 58%. In Habermalz's report of 44 treated lesions, no responses were seen in eleven cases treated with fraction sizes of ≤ 5 Gy. Seventeen of 33 complete responders were seen among those treated with fraction sizes of 6 Gy or greater.[28] Unfortunately, the size of the lesion was not analyzed in this study, nor was the relationship of fraction size and total dose well discussed. Hornsey's report of combined data from the United

Kingdom and Australia on 94 lesions treated with various fractionation schemes stated that only 20–23% of patients treated with fraction sizes less than 3 Gy showed a "good response" (undefined), whereas 50–60% were good responders to fractions of 3-8 Gy.[36] Once again, however, tumor size was not evaluated. In Konefal's report of 67 measurable lesions, fraction size of ≤ 5 Gy resulted in only 9% complete response. Fractions > 5 Gy had 50% complete response.[42] In this last report, for lesions less than 3 cm in size, fraction size retained its significance in determining complete response rate (54% vs 15% for > 5 Gy fraction sizes vs ≤ 5 Gy).

Although each of these studies lends support to the notion that larger fraction sizes have a greater effect on melanoma than standard fraction sizes, the retrospective nature of these studies weakens the strength of the argument for a uniformly improved response to larger fraction sizes.[70,71] Each study included a marked heterogeneity of tumor sizes and locations, with no prospective attempt to compare various fractionation schemes. One major concern not adequately addressed centers on the possibility that inadequate total doses were used in cases where small fraction sizes were utilized. Logically, one could assume that patients with more extensive fields would be treated with smaller fraction sizes. Total doses for a large portion of cases therefore may have been lower than those which might have been utilized if the aim was not limited to palliation. A major review by Trott et al failed to show any improvement with the use of fraction sizes > 4 Gy.[70,71]

The only prospective trial that has compared two different fractionation schemes for measurable melanoma lesions was the randomized Phase III trial carried out by the RTOG(RTOG 83-05) and reported in 1991.[59] One hundred thirty-seven patients were stratified according to tumor size ($\leq$ 5 cm or > 5 cm) and location (soft tissue, nodal or other site), and randomized to receive either 4 fractions of 8 Gy in three weeks or 20 fractions of 2.5 Gy in four weeks. Complete response rates were comparable (24.2% vs. 23.4%), as were partial response rates (35.5% vs 34.4%), with no significant differences seen in either the smaller or larger lesions. (Table 2) For lesions < 5 cm, the complete response rate was higher, although it did not achieve statistical significance. Both schedules were well tolerated although there was a slight increase in skin toxicity (ulceration) noted in the larger fraction arm.

Table 2. RTOG83–05: Malignant Melanoma Response by Treatment & Lesion Size[59]

Treatment	<5 cm>		>5 cm	
	PR	CR	PR	CR
4 x 8.0 GY	18.0%	33.3%	48.6%	17.1%
20 x 2.5 GY	28.6%	28.6%	38.9%	19.4%

The resolution to the apparent contradictions surrounding the early radiobiologic data and the apparent equivalence of small and large fractionation schemes seen in a randomized study may be found in review done by Rofstad.[56] Survival curve parameters were reviewed for 46 separate melanoma cell lines (from established cell lines, disaggregated xenografts, and disaggregated surgical specimens). The most significant observation was that different melanoma lines, both in vitro and in vivo exhibited widespread irradiation sensitivities, from a level of sensitivity approaching that of the most radioresponsive tumors known (lymphoma and neuroblastoma) to a degree of resistance akin to the notoriously radio-nonresponsive osteosarcoma and glioblastoma cell lines. Furthermore, cell subpopulations from a single patient or cell line may have different radiosensitivities.

The linear-quadratic (LQ) formula, $SF = e^{-\alpha D - \beta D^2}$, was derived as an attempt to explain the shape of the initial portion of the cell-survival curve found in fractionated radiation experiments.[21,22,23,69,74] "α" represents the linear non-repairable component of cell-kill, "ß" represents the more efficient component of cell-kill after repair capability has been exceeded. The ratio of $\alpha/\text{ß}$ gives that dose at which the two components are roughly equal, and is also an inverse measure of the repair capacity of a given cell line. In analyzing the $\alpha/\text{ß}$ ratios for these melanoma cell lines, Rofstad discovered a wide range of values. Nineteen of 46 cell lines had an $\alpha/\text{ß}$ ratio of < 5 Gy, levels similar to those of late responding tissues.[56] For these particular cell lines, a larger individual fraction size would be necessary to obtain a discernible effect, and overall treatment times would be of only minor importance. These melanomas would be compatible with the clinical observations of Overgaard and others.[27,36,49,51] The remaining 27 of 46 cell lines had $\alpha/\text{ß}$ ratios above the limit for late responding tissues, more akin to the $\alpha/\text{ß}$ ratios for the majority of tumors, suggesting that these lines might actually benefit from the use of smaller individual fractions for a higher overall dose. The conclusions of Rofstad's analyses are that melanomas may differ significantly in the responsiveness to radiation from patient to patient, and even from lesion to lesion in a single patient. Whereas some tumors might be expected to respond best to large fractions, others might well benefit from hyperfractionated regimens.

The development of in vitro predictive assays for assessment of radiation responsiveness would be critical for the selection of appropriate fractionation schemes. Work is currently being done with assays of tumor kinetics using flow cytometry techniques on biopsy samples of tumors from individual patients, such as potential doubling time (T_{pot}) and IUdR/BUdR labelling indices (LI).[6] Early results from a clinical trial in Europe suggest that such assays may accurately predict which tumors may benefit from an altered fractionation scheme.[6] Another approach has looked at the surviving fraction of melanoma xenografts after treatment with a single fraction of 2 Gy in vitro (SF_2). A positive correlation has been found between the SF_2 and the inherent radiocurability of these tumors in vivo.[57] This approach is currently being evaluated in clinical trials with head and neck and cervical carcinomas.[57] Until such time as these assays are proven to be of clinical use and are readily available, the clinician is left with the dilemma of determining the appropriate fractionation scheme. The choice of schedule should be based upon assessment of the patient's overall current status, extent of disease, tumor characteristics, and prolonged outlook of the patient, as well as the risk of damage to local late reacting tissues which might result from large dose-per-fraction radiation schemes.

RADIATION AS A PRIMARY MODALITY

Surgery remains the cornerstone of therapy for localized melanoma. There are, however, certain conditions where a surgical approach might not be desirable, and alternative therapy must be considered. Cases in which the patient is not a good surgical candidate, refuses surgery or would require very extensive resections and grafts not warranted due to the poor overall prognosis might best be served with the use of definitive radiotherapy.

LENTIGO MALIGNA

Lentigo maligna (LM or Hutchinson's melanotic freckle) is a distinct entity characterized by a slowly progressive pigmented lesion usually involving patches of skin on the head and neck in elderly patients.[33] The lesion is confined to the epidermis. If unattended, up to one half of these will progressive to invasive melanoma (termed lentigo maligna melanoma, or LMM),[29,33,39] and ten percent will metastasize. If possible, therefore, resection is considered the primary approach to preinvasive lentigo maligna. Given the advanced age of the patient, however, and the extent of the lesion in some cases, a surgical approach is not always suitable. Radiation therapy has long been in use in Europe using a number of techniques, including the Miescher technique (contact radiotherapy technique with 50% depth dose at 1 mm, delivering doses up

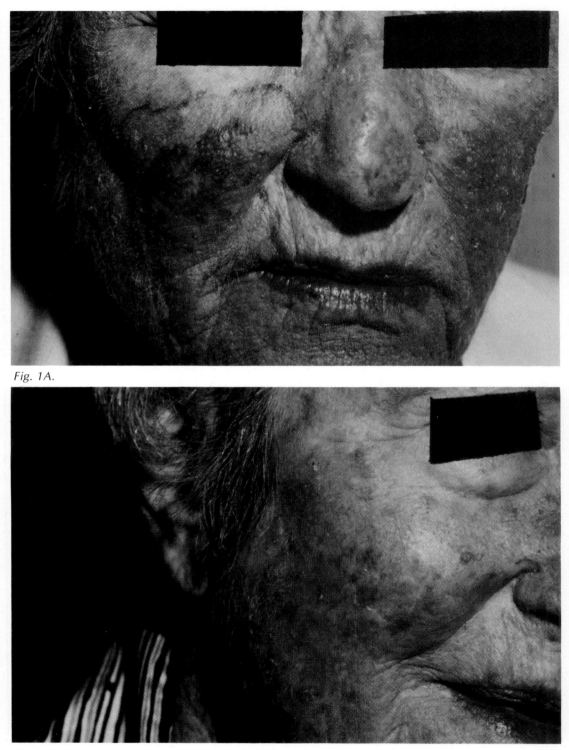

Fig. 1A.

Fig. 1B.

Fig. 1. Lentigo maligna on the cheek of a 76-year-old female, A) at initiation of radiation treatment and B) six months after completion of radiation.

10,000 cGy in 4–5 treatments) with satisfactory results.[66] As Harwood has pointed out, any appreciable thickness of these lesions makes this technique undesirable due to the extremely rapid dose drop-off in tissue.[29] Several reports from Princess Margaret Hospital on the use of more penetrating orthovoltage therapy for LM have yielded excellent results.[29,31,32,33,35] One hundred to 280 KeV orthovoltage units were used to deliver a dose to the lesion plus a 1 cm margin. Appropriate lead shielding was designed to spare local uninvolved areas, especially the eyes and lips. Doses were tailored to the size of the lesions (1–2.9 cm diameter are treated with 3500 cGy in 5 fractions; 3–4.9 cm diameter lesions with 4500 cGy in 10 fractions; ≥ 5 cm diameter lesions with 5000 cGy in 15–20 fractions). Using this technique, local control was obtained in 18 of 20 patients with LM followed for a median of 26 months with an excellent cosmetic outcome. (Figs. 1A, B) The median time to complete response was approximately 7–8 months, with some requiring up to 24 months until complete regression was noted.

LENTIGO MALIGNA MELANOMA

Patients with lentigo maligna melanoma also have been treated with definitive radiotherapy using similar dosing schedules. (Table 3) Harwood reported that 21 of 23 patients with LMM had tumor control by irradiation with follow-up ranging from 1 month to 7 years.[29,30] Elsmann treated 60 invasive melanomas, the majority being LMM, with superficial radiation (30–100 kVp) after either biopsy or subtotal resection of the nodular

component.[18] There was only one in-field recurrence noted, with follow-up ranging from 0–170 months (median 42 months). No difference in response rate was noted for those treated with large individual fractions or standard fraction sizes. Radiation therapy should be seriously considered as an alternative to surgery in circumstances where a considerable cosmetic deficit would result in a large skin graft.

Table 3. Radiation Therapy for Lentigo Maligna Melanoma

Author	Ref.	#	LC	Median Fu
Harwood	9	23	90%	26 months
Elsmann	18	64	98%	42 months

NODULAR MELANOMA

Little information is available on the effectiveness of radiation therapy for primary superficial spreading melanoma or nodular melanoma. In a report from Toronto on nodular melanoma, 5 of 9 patients treated with the "0–7–21" approach (800 cGy delivered on day zero, seven and twenty-one) for gross residual disease after attempted resection of nodular melanoma had complete responses with short follow-up of 7–42 months.[39] Surgery is unquestionably the recommended approach to these lesions, but radiation therapy must be considered in cases where surgery is not feasible or the resection is incomplete. (Figs. 2A, B)

MUCOSAL MELANOMA

Mucosal melanomas, arising in the nasal cavity, paranasal sinuses, oral cavity,

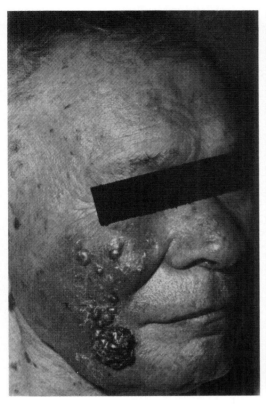

Fig. 2A.

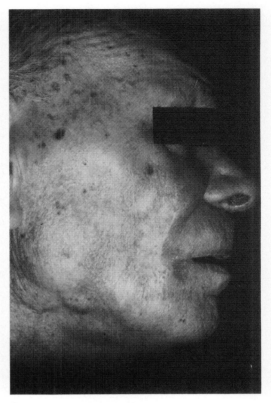

Fig. 2B.

Fig. 2. Localized nodular melanoma, A) prior to radiation therapy and B) six months after completion of radiation.

anorectal region, cervix, vagina and vulva, constitute approximately 1–3% of all melanomas.[34,37,38,46,75] The overall prognosis is very poor, with most series reporting five-year survivals of only 10–18%. For head and neck melanomas, radical excision is the commonly recommended approach, but local recurrence has been reported in up to 60% of cases treated with excision alone.[24,38] Following a policy of wide local excision with adjuvant radiation used routinely for gross or microscopic residual disease, Stern from M. D. Anderson has reported a five-year DFS of 40% in 42 patients.[65] In most reports,

however, the majority of patients die of systemic disease, with or without components of local failure. Given the dismal prognosis and the extent of aggressive surgery often required, consideration has been given to the use of definitive radiation as an alternate approach. In a combined total of 79 patients treated with a variety of radiation schedules with curative intent for mucosal melanomas of the head and neck, a cumulative 71% initial complete response was seen.[7,24,25,34] (Table 4) Overall, 48% of patients retained control of the primary site for the duration of followup or until death.

Little information has been published about the role of radiation in the treatment of vulvovaginal or anorectal melanomas, as extensive surgical resections are standardly performed.[12,46,75] Given the overall poor prognosis of these cases, and extrapolating from the information regarding radiation's effectiveness in head and neck sites, it is reasonable to consider high dose radiation as an alternative to exenterative surgery.

CHOROIDAL MELANOMA

Melanoma involving the choroid of the eye deserves special attention. Lesions of the choroid are often associated with changes in vision at a relatively early stage, or detected on routine fundoscopic exam in the asymptomatic patient. Tumors are separated into three categories based on their size.[9,63] Melanocytic lesions measuring less than 10 mm in maximum diameter and less than 3 mm in height are categorized as "small". Close observation is justified as the initial approach to these lesions if there are no signs of activity such as subretinal fluid accumulation. In some reports, up to 59% of these will not be progressive over a 5-year period.[63] Any

evidence of growth on serial examination requires prompt therapeutic intervention. Medium-sized lesions (3–5 mm in height, 10–15 mm in base diameter) and large choroidal melanomas (> 5 mm in height, > 15 mm in base diameter) require prompt intervention. Standard therapy for these lesions in the past was enucleation. Over the last decade, however, a major shift has occurred towards eye preservation therapy, using either charged particle irradiation (protons, helium ions) or episcleral plaque radiotherapy (^{125}I, ^{60}Co, ^{106}Ru, ^{103}Pd).

A nationwide prospective protocol, the Collaborative Ocular Melanoma Study (COMS) is currently underway randomizing patients to plaque radiotherapy versus enucleation.[60] Results of this study will not be available for a number of years. In the meantime, single institutional reviews of plaque experience have shown excellent levels of local control. In a series of 1,016 patients treated at Will's Eye Hospital with plaque radiotherapy, only 6% required enucleation for either tumor regrowth or radiation complications such as severe neovascular glaucoma.[63] Of 235 patients treated with ^{125}I plaques at UCSF, an actuarial local control of 82% at five

Table 4. Radiotherapy for Mucosal Melanoma of the Head and Neck

1st Author	Ref.	No. of Patients	CR Rate	Local Control
Harwood & Cummings	4	24	72%	44%
Berthelsen	7	14	57%	36%
Gaze	24	13	62%	38%
Gilligan	25	28	79%	61%

years has been reported, with a 12% risk of distant metastases.[54]

The results with both proton and helium ions have been equally encouraging, although the number of sites capable of delivering this therapy are quite limited. In a group of 556 patients treated with protons at the Harvard Cyclotron, between 1975 and 1984, 16% developed distant metastases, with an overall survival rate comparable to those patients treated by enucleation.[61] A later update on local control rates in 1006 patients treated at the same facility showed a 1.2% incidence of documented local recurrence and a 0.3% incidence of apparent second melanomas in the same eye.[48] At five years, the risk of enucleation was 10%, with 4.6% performed for neovascular glaucoma, 2.5% for tumor regrowth and 2.8% for other treatment related complications.[17] Overall, there was a 5-year local control rate of 96.3%.

Helium ion beams have been used in the treatment of choroidal melanomas since 1978 at the Lawrence Berkeley Laboratory.[43] In a report of 307 patients treated, the actuarial 5- and 10-year local control was 96%. The 5-year actuarial determinate survival was 81% and 75% at 10 years. At five years the rate of enucleation was 17%, 2% for local recurrence and 15% for neovascular glaucoma-related complications.

It is not yet apparent that either plaque therapy or charged particle therapy is superior. In a prospective randomized study comparing helium ions versus ^{125}I plaque therapy for medium-sized lesions at UCSF, overall survival was not different and the enucleation rates were comparable at 7.7% and 5.6% respectively.[11] This study has now been closed, and final results are pending. Both plaque therapy and charged particle therapy appear to be equivalent to enucleation in terms of overall survival, and have the obvious advantages of retention of the eye and preservation of useful vision in some cases. At five years, visual acuity better than 20/200 is maintained in 40–60% of patients treated with these modalities.[10,17,44] Gradual visual deterioration over a period of several years will be seen, however, in a significant proportion of the patients treated with radiation, either charged particle or plaque therapy, due to the development of radiation retinopathy, cataracts, and neovascular glaucoma. Visual loss is a function of proximity of tumor to the fovea and optic disc, size of the tumor, and dose delivered.[10,17,44] Hyperthermia in conjunction with radiotherapy is currently being evaluated as a means of lowering the dose of radiation necessary to control tumor and lowering the incidence of visual deterioration.[20,68]

RADIATION THERAPY AS AN ADJUVANT TO SURGERY

Local resection of nonulcerated melanomas with thickness < 1.5 mm is associated with an excellent 5-year survival rate (84–100% in various studies), and a local-regional relapse rate of 20%, according to data from the World Health Organization.[4,72] Although the routine use of elective lymph node dissection in stage I patients has not been proven to be warranted, elective lymph node dissection in patients at high risk for regional recurrence such as those with thickness > 4 mm or the presence of ulceration may be justified given the 40% risk of local-regional relapse in these cases.[72] There is, however, no consensus as yet regarding the benefit of this approach.[3] An alternative to lymph node dissection for these cases was proposed by Ang.[1] Thirty-five stage I patients who presented with primary lesions ≥ 1.5 mm or Clark's level ≥ III were treated with wide local excision and elective irradiation of draining lymph nodes as well as the tumor bed, using a hypofractionated regimen, i.e. 6 Gy per fraction times 5 in 2.5 weeks. With a median followup of 15 months, 2-year actuarial locoregional control was 95%, and 2-year crude survival was 80%, a substantial reduction from the 40% local-regional relapse rate reported by the World Health Organization.[72] It is, however, unclear that radiation therapy would be equivalent to prophylactic node dissection in cases at high risk of local-regional relapse.

The role of adjuvant therapy in Stage II patients remains to be elucidated as well. Surgical resection of patients who present with clinically suspicious lymph nodes has resulted in an overall survival rate of 27–42%.[8,13,47,53] Distant metastases remain the main cause of death, as we await the development of more successful systemic therapy. Patient survival, however, is not the only consideration. Local-regional failure may have a profound impact on quality of life and needs to be addressed. Patients with tumor penetrating the lymph node capsule, multiple involved lymph nodes, nodes ≥ 3 cm in size, or those who only had a positive lymph node biopsy have an increased risk of regional as well as distant failure.[32,39] Johansson reported the use of the previously described "0–7–21" regimen of radiation for patients such as these, with

26 of 30 showing no evidence of recurrence.[39] Ang et al from the M. D. Anderson Cancer Center reported 48 patients who were treated with either pr-operative (6 Gy x 4) or postoperative radiotherapy (6 Gy x 5 in two and a half weeks) for previously untreated stage II disease or limited nodal relapse after prior primary excision).[1] Three-year actuarial local control for these groups was 83–90%, with three-year crude survival rates of 69–71%. In this study any patient with stage II disease or isolated nodal relapse was treated, and no attempt was made to differentiate those at greatest risk for recurrence. The only prospective randomized therapy of adjuvant radiation therapy in stage II patients was reported by Creagan et al at the Mayo Clinic.[14] This was a small study of 56 analyzable cases which were stratified for disease status (untreated primary, local disease on control, unknown primary), but not for thickness, level of invasion, presence of ulceration or number of nodes involved. Patients were randomized to either postlymphadenectomy irradiation (daily dose of 178 cGy to 25 Gy, followed by a 3-week break; then followed by an additional 25 Gy) or observation. No significant differences were noted in either local-regional control or overall survival. This study suffers from a lack of complete stratification and the use of an unconventional radiation therapy regimen. The question of the value of adjuvant radiation therapy to regional lymphatic beds in patients with poor risk stage II disease remains unanswered. The RTOG is currently planning a Phase III randomized study building upon the M.D. Anderson Cancer Center experience to address this question.

Table 5. Radiotherapy of Brain Metastases from Malignant Melanoma

1st Author	Ref.	No. of Patients	Median Survival (Mos.)	% Improved
Katz	40	29 single	3.2	62
		23 multiple	2.2	30
Strauss	67	20	—	50
Vlock	73	46	3.0	37
Ziegler and Cooper	76	72	4.6	62
Konefel	42	23	—	39

RADIATION THERAPY FOR METASTATIC MELANOMA

The palliative role for radiation therapy in metastatic melanoma is well established despite continued dispute over the optimal fractionation scheme as discussed earlier. The reports by Habermalz,[28] Hornsey[36] and the RTOG[59] illustrated that response rates in excess of 50% can be expected for soft tissue and nodal metastases with up to 47% being completely responsive. As suggested by the RTOG trial results, it would appear that either large fractions or standard fraction schemes are equally successful in achieving responses in metastatic sites.

Cerebral metastases of melanoma are associated with a median survival ranging from two to six months.[55,76] Response rates

Table 6. Radiotherapy ± Hyperthermia for Malignant Melanoma*

1st Author	Ref.	CR Rate (%)	
		RT	RT + Heat
Arcangelli	2	53	76
Perez	52	24	59
Kim	41	46	69
Overgaard	50	61	90

*Advanced, recurrent or metastatic

range from 30% to 62%. (Table 5) In several retrospective studies of the effectiveness of radiation for cerebral metastases, no significant advantage was seen to high dose per fraction over standard fractionation with 300 cGy x 10.[55,76] The only group that showed an improved overall survival was that group in which isolated CNS metastases were identified and resected prior to whole brain irradiation.[55] In this subgroup, median survival was extended to thirteen months.

Few reports are available on the effectiveness of radiation for spinal cord compression by melanoma. In a series of 17 patients with epidural compression due to melanoma, a response rate of 71% was observed, with no discernible difference with respect to various fractionation schemes.[55] Bone metastases have a higher response rate than lesions within the CNS in most series, ranging from 50% to 85%. Once again, dose per fraction does not appear to be a critical determinant of response.

Hyperthermia has been investigated extensively over the past few decades as an adjuvant to both radiotherapy and chemotherapy in the treatment of melanoma.[62,64] (Fig. 2) By itself, heat is cytotoxic to tumor cells. This cytotoxicity is aided by conditions of chronic hypoxia, acidic pH and decreased nutritional supply, conditions commonly found within poorly vascularized tumors. In addition, heat acts as a potentiator of radiation by interfering with radiation repair mechanisms, and by enhancing cell kill in the relatively radioresistant portion of the cell cycle (S-phase).[16,45] Melanoma lends itself well to investigation of the effectiveness of hyperthermia due to the superficial nature of metastatic lesions which make it technically more feasible to deliver adequate heat treatments. In addition, early studies suggesting that melanoma survival curves had a broad shoulder indicating increase sublethal damage repair supported the investigation of hyperthermia as a possible means of interfering with this repair. The technical aspects of hyperthermia are beyond the scope of this chapter, and the interested reader is referred to the excellent review by Perez et al.[52] A limited number of clinical reports dealing specifically with hyperthermia and radiotherapy in the treatment of melanomas have been released.[2,19,26,41,45,50,58,62] Each of these reports suggested an increase of complete response rate when hyperthermia was added to external beam radiation therapy. (Table 6) Emami reported a complete response rate of 59% in 49 patients treated with combined heat and radiation.[19] Overgaard reported a 56% complete response rate among 102 lesions treated.[50] Gonzalez reported a 50% complete response rate in 28 lesions.[26] It is seen from these reports that hyperthermia, when delivered appropriately, can improve the response rate for soft tissue metastases associated with metastatic melanoma. (Figs. 3A,B)

SUMMARY

The antiquated notion of melanoma as a radiation resistant tumor has no place in the current management of this devastating illness. Surgery remains the cornerstone of management of this disease, with the possible exception of choroidal melanoma. The use of radiation as an adjuvant in patients at high risk of local-regional recurrence after resection, or as a

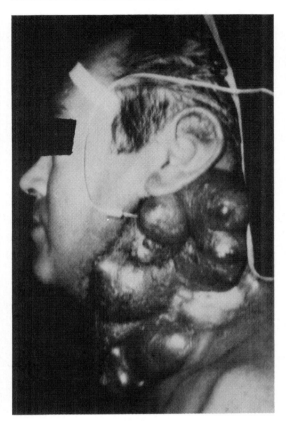

primary modality in those who are not appropriate candidates for major surgery must be considered. The use of rapid assays of tumor intrinsic cellular radiosensitivity and proliferative kinetic parameters may prove to be useful in determining the optimal radiation therapy schedule for the individual patient. As we await the development of more effective systemic therapy, attention must be given to improving local-regional control. There can be no cure without local-regional control. Radiation therapy, in addition to surgery, plays an important role in achieving local-regional control.

Fig. 3. Massive nodal recurrence of melanoma, A) prior to initiation of combined external beam radiation and microwave hyperthermia [single thermometry probe in tumor] and B) after completion of hyperthermia, radiation and neck dissection.

Fig. 3A.

Fig. 3B.

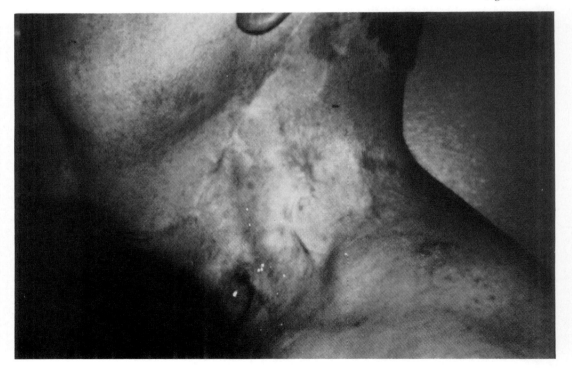

References

1. Ang KK, Byers RM, Peters LJ et al. Regional radiotherapy as adjuvant treatment for head and neck malignant melanoma. Preliminary results. Arch Otolaryngol Head Neck Surg 1990; 116:169-72.

2. Arcangeli G, Benassi M, Cividalli A et al. Radiotherapy and hyperthermia. Analysis of clinical results and identification of prognostic variables. Cancer 1987; 60:950-6.

3. Balch CM. The role of elective lymph node dissection in melanoma: Rationale, results and controversies. Journal of Clinical Oncology 1988; 6:163-72.

4. Balch CM, Soong SJ, Shaw HM. A comparison of worldwide melanoma data. In: Balch CM, Milton GH, eds. Cutaneous Melanoma. Philadelphia: J. B. Lippincott, 1985:507-18.

5. Barranco SC, Romsdahl MM, Humphrey RM. The radiation response of human malignant melanoma cells grown in vitro. Cancer Res 1971; 31:830-3.

6. Begg AC, Hofland I, Van Glabekke M et al. Predictive value of potential doubling time for radiotherapy of head and neck tumor patients: results from the EORTC Cooperative Trial 22851. Seminars in Radiation Oncology 1992; 2:22-5.

7. Berthelsen A, Andersen AP, Jensen TS, Hansen HS. Melanomas of the mucosa in the oral cavity and the upper respiratory passages. Cancer 1984; 54:907-12.

8. Callery C, Cochran AJ, Roe DJ et al. Factors prognostic for survival in patients with malignant melanoma spread to the regional lymph nodes. Ann Surg 1982; 196:69-75.

9. Char DH. Clinical Ocular Oncology. New York: Churchill Livingston, 1989.

10. Char DH. Current treatments and trials in uveal melanoma. Oncology 1989; 3:113-21.

11. Char DH, Castro JR, Quivey JM et al. Uveal melanoma radiation. 125I brachytherapy versus helium ion irradiation. Ophthalmology 1989; 96:1708-15.

12. Chung AF, Casey MJ, Flannery JT et al. Malignant melanoma of the vagi, 1980.

13. Coit DG, Rogatko A, Brennan MF. Prognostic factors in patients with melanoma metastatic to axillary or inguinal lymph nodes. A multivariate analysis. Ann Surg 1991; 214:627-36.

14. Creagan ET, Cupps RE, Ivins JC et al. Adjuvant radiation therapy for regional nodal metastases from malignant melanoma: a randomized, prospective study. Cancer 1978; 42:2206-10.

15. Dewey DL. The radiosensitivity of melanoma cells in culture. Br J Radiol 1971; 44:816-7.

16. Dewey WC. Mechanisms of thermal injury and thermal radiosensitization. In: Sugahara T, Saito M, eds, Hyperthermic Oncology. London: Taylor and Francis, 1989:7580.

17. Egan KM, Gragoudas ES, Seddon J Mea. The risk of enucleation after proton beam irradiation of uveal melanoma. Ophthalmology 1989; 96:1377-83.

18. Elsmann HJ, Ernst K, Suter L. Radiotherapy of primary human melanomas-experiences and suggestions. Strahlenther Onkol 1991; 167:387-91.

19. Emami B, Perez CA, Konefal J et al. Thermoradiotherapy of malignant melanoma. Int J Hyperthermia 1988; 4:373-81.

20. Finger PT, Packer S, Paglione RW et al. Thermoradiotherapy of choroidal melanoma. Clinical experience. Ophthalmology 1989; 96:1384-8.

21. Fowler JF. Fractionated radiation therapy after Strandqvist. Acta Radiologica — Oncology 1984; 23:209-16.

22. Fowler JF. The linear quadratic formula and progress in fractionated radiotherapy. British Journal of Radiology 1989; 62:679-94.

23. Fowler JF. Radiobiologic principles in fractionated radiotherapy. Seminars in Radiation Oncology 1992; 2:16-21.

24. Gaze MN, Kerr GR, Smyth JF. Mucosal melanomas of the head and neck: The Scottish experience. The Scottish

Melanoma Group. Clin Oncol (R Coll Radiol) 1990; 2:277-83.

25. Gilligan D, Slevin NJ. Radical radiotherapy for 28 cases of mucosal melanoma of the nasal cavity and sinuses. British Journal of Radiology 1991; 64:1147-50.

26. Gonzalez GD, van DJD, Blank LE, Rumke P. Combined treatment with radiation and hyperthermia in metastatic malignant melanoma. Radiother Oncol 1986; 6:105-13.

27. Habermalz HJ. Irradiation of malignant melanoma: experience in the past and present [editorial]. Int J Radiat Oncol Biol Phys 1981; 7:131-3.

28. Habermalz HJ, Fischer JJ. Radiation therapy of malignant melanoma: experience with high individual treatment doses. Cancer 1976; 38:2258-62.

29. Harwood AR. Conventional radiotherapy in the treatment of lentigo maligna and lentigo maligna melanoma. J Am Acad Dermatol 1982; 6:310-6.

30. Harwood AR. Conventional fractionated radiotherapy for 51 patients with lentigo maligna and lentigo maligna melanoma. Int J Radiat Oncol Biol Phys 1983; 9:1019-21.

31. Harwood AR. Malignant melanoma: the myth of radioresistance [letter]. Can J Surg 1983; 26:14.

32. Harwood AR. Melanomas of the head and neck. J Otolaryngol 1983; 12:64-9.

33. Harwood AR, Cummings BJ. Radiotherapy for malignant melanoma: a re-appraisal. Cancer Treat Rev 1981; 8:271-82.

34. Harwood AR, Cummings BJ. Radiotherapy for mucosal melanomas. Int J Radiat Oncol Biol Phys 1982; 8:1121-6.

35. Harwood AR, Lawson VG. Radiation therapy for melanomas of the head and neck. Head Neck Surg 1982; 4:468-74.

36. Hornsey S. The relationship between total dose, number of fractions and fractions size in the response of malignant melanoma in patients. Br J Radiol 1978; 51:905-9.

37. Hoyt DJ, Jordan T, Fisher SR. Mucosal melanoma of the head and neck. Arch Otolaryngol Head Neck Surg 1989; 115:1096-9.

38. Iversen K, Robins RE. Mucosal malignant melanomas. Am J Surg 1980; 139:660-4.

39. Johansson CR, Harwood AR, Cummings BJ, Quirt I. 0-7-21 radiotherapy in nodular melanoma. Cancer 1983; 51:226-32.

40. Katz H, Redding KG. Therapeutic challenge of premalignant and malignant skin lesions. Geriatrics 1975; 30:53-6.

41. Kim JH, Hahn EW, Ahmed SA. Combination hyperthermia and radiation therapy for malignant melanoma. Cancer 1982; 50:478-82.

42. Konefal JB, Emami B, Pilepich MV. Malignant melanoma: analysis of dose fractionation in radiation therapy. Radiology 1987; 164:607-10.

43. Linstadt D, Castro J, Char D et al. Longterm results of helium ion irradiation of uveal melanoma. Int J Radiat Oncol Biol Phys 1990; 19:613-8.

44. Linstadt D, Char DH, Castro JR et al. Vision following helium ion radiotherapy of uveal melanoma: a Northern California Oncology Group study. Int J Radiat Oncol Biol Phys 1988; 15:347-52.

45. Mameghan H, Knittel T. Response of melanoma to heat and radiation therapy—a review of the literature and experience from The Prince of Wales Hospital, Sydney. Med J Aust 1988; 149:474-6.

46. McKinnon JG, Kokal WA, Neifeld JP, Kay S. Natural history and treatment of mucosal melanoma. J Surg Oncol 1989; 41:222-5.

47. Morton DL, Wanek L, Nizze JA et al. Improved long-term survival after lymphadenectomy of melanoma metastatic to regional nodes. Analysis of prognostic factors in 1134 patients from the John Wayne Cancer Clinic. Ann Surg 1991; 214:491-9.

48. Munzenrider JE, Verhey LJ, Gragoudas ES et al. Conservative treatment of uveal melanoma: local recurrence after proton

beam therapy. Int J Radiat Oncol Biol Phys 1989; 17:493-8.

49. Overgaard J. The role of radiotherapy in recurrent and metastatic malignant melanoma: a clinical radiobiological study. Int J Radiat Oncol Biol Phys 1989; 12:867-72.

50. Overgaard J, Overgaard M. Hyperthermia as an adjuvant to radiotherapy in the treatment of malignant melanoma. Int J Hyperthermia 1987; 3:483-501.

51. Overgaard J, Overgaard M, Hansen PV, von dMH. Some factors of importance in the radiation treatment of malignant melanoma. Radiother Oncol 1986; 5:183-92.

52. Perez CA, Emami B, Myerson RJ, Roti JL. Hyperthermia. In: Perez CA, Brady LW, eds. Principles and Practice of Radiation Oncology. Philadelphia: J. B. Lippincott, 1992:396-446.

53. Presant CA, Bartolucci AA. Prognostic factors in metastatic malignant melanoma: The Southeastern Cancer Study Group Experience. Cancer 1982; 49:2192-6.

54. Quivey JM, Char DH, Phillips T. High intensity 125-Iodine plaque treatment of uveal melanoma. ASTRO, Washington DC, 1991:181-182.

55. Rate WR, Solin LJ, Turrisi AT. Palliative radiotherapy for metastatic malignant melanoma: brain metastases, bone metastases, and spinal cord compression. Int J Radiat Oncol Biol Phys 1988; 15:859-64.

56. Rofstad EK. Radiation biology of malignant melanoma. Acta Radiol [Oncol] 1986; 25:1-10.

57. Rofstad EK. Influence of cellular radiation sensitivity on local tumor control of human melanoma xenografts given fractionated radiation treatment. Cancer Res 1991; 51:4609-12.

58. Rofstad EK, Brustad T. Differences in thermosensitization among cloned cell lines isolated from a single human melanoma xenograft. Radiat Res 1986; 106:147-55.

59. Sause WT, Cooper JS, Rush S et al. Fraction size in external beam radiation therapy in the treatment of melanoma. Int J Radiat Oncol Biol Phys 1991; 20:429-32.

60. Schachat AP. Collaborative ocular melanoma study. In: Ryan SJ, eds. Retina. St. Louis: C. V. Mosby, 1989:733-6.

61. Seddon JM, Gragoudas ES, Egan KM et al. Relative survival rates after alternative therapies for uveal melanoma. Ophthalmology 1990; 97:769-77.

62. Shidnia H, Hornback NB, Shen RN et al. An overview of the role of radiation therapy and hyperthermia in treatment of malignant melanoma. Adv Exp Med Biol 1990; 267:531-45.

63. Shields JA, Shields CL. Management of posterior uveal melanoma. In: Shields JA, Shields CL, eds. Intraocular Tumors. Philadelphia: W. B. Saunders, 1992:1712-6.

64. Sneed PK, Phillips TL. Combining hyperthermia and radiation: how beneficial? Oncology 1991; 5:99-108.

65. Stern SJ, Guillamondegui OM. Mucosal melanoma of the head and neck. Head Neck 1991; 13:22-7.

66. Storck H, Ott F, Schwarz K. Maligne melanome. In: Zuppinger A, Krowkowski E, eds. Encyclopedia of Medical Radiology. Heidelburg: Springer, 1972:161-257.

67. Strauss A, Dritschilo A, Nathanson L, Piro AJ. Radiation therapy of malignant melanomas: an evaluation of clinically used fractionation schemes. Cancer 1981; 47:1262-6.

68. Swift PS, Stauffer PR, Fries PDea. Microwave hyperthermia for choroidal melanoma in rabbits. Investigative Ophthalmology and Visual Science 1990; 31:1754-60.

69. Thames HD, Bentzen SM, Turesson I, et al. Time-dose factors in radiotherapy: a review of the human data. Radiotherapy and Oncology 1990; 19:219-35.

70. Trott KR. The optimal radiation dose per fraction for the treatment of malignant melanomas [editorial]. Int J Radiat Oncol Biol Phys 1991; 20:905-7.

71. Trott KR, von LH, Kummermehr J. The radiosensitivity of malignant

melanomas part I: experimental studies. Int J Radiat Oncol Biol Phys 1981; 7:9-13.

72. Veronesi U. Metastatic spread of stage I melanoma of the skin. Tumori 1983; 69:449-54.

73. Vlock DR, Kirkwood JM, Leutzinger C, Kapp DSea. High dose fraction radiotherapy for intracranial metastases of malignant melanoma. Cancer1982; 49:2289-94.

74. Williams MV, Denekamp J, Fowler JF. A review of alpha/beta ratios for experimental tumors: implications for clinical studies of altered fractionation. International Journal of Radiation Oncology, Biology and Physics 1985: 11:87-96.

75. Wong JH, Cagle LA, Storm FK, Morton DL. Natural history of surgically treated mucosal melanoma. Am J Surg 1987; 154:54-7.

76. Ziegler JC, Cooper JS. Brain metastases from malignant melanoma: conventional vs. high-dose-per-fraction radiotherapy. Int J Radiat Oncol Biol Phys 1986; 12:1839-42.

CHAPTER 7

CHEMOTHERAPY
OF ADVANCED MELANOMA

Charles W. Taylor
and Evan M. Hersh

This discussion will focus on use of chemotherapeutic agents as therapy for patients with malignant melanoma that has progressed beyond the primary tumor site and/or regional lymph nodes to involve distant metastatic sites. Such patients have stage III disease according to the previous three-stage system[1] or stage IV disease as defined by the newer American Joint Committee on Cancer (AJCC) staging system.[2] Although the majority of patients with melanoma present with early stage disease that can potentially be cured by surgical resection, those who develop metastatic disease have an extremely poor prognosis. The median survival for patients with only one site of melanoma metastasis is seven months.[3] The incidence of melanoma is increasing[4] and in 1991 an estimated 6,500 new cases were diagnosed.[5]

The five year survival rates for patients with malignant melanoma vary dramatically according to extent of disease: localized disease – 90% five year survival, regional involvement – 55%, distant metastases – 14%.[5] The most common first sites of distant metastasis are skin, subcutaneous tissues, and distant lymph nodes, followed in order of decreasing frequency by lung, brain, liver and bone.[6] Patients with isolated lung metastases have the longest survival duration (median – 11.4 months) followed by skin/subcutaneous tissue/distant lymph nodes (7.2 months), bone (6.0 months), brain (5.0 months) and liver (2.4 months).[3] The two most important prognostic factors for survival of patients with metastatic melanoma are visceral versus non-visceral disease (p > 0.001) and 1 versus 2 versus 3 or more sites of metastatic disease (p = 0.0001).[3]

Despite improved response rates in recent years, chemotherapy for metastatic melanoma does not result in consistent survival benefit. Thus, rational interpretation of results from chemotherapy trials for patients with metastatic melanoma must consider prognostic factors in the patient population studied. Joensuu recently reported a 16% response rate in 55 patients with disseminated malignant melanoma treated with DTIC (dacarbazine) and CCNU (lomustine) and observed an association between chemotherapy response and rate of disease progression.[7] The responding patients survived longer than non-responding patients but also had a longer time interval from diagnosis to development of distant metastases and a longer survival after disease progression on chemotherapy. This suggests that the natural history of metastatic melanoma varies in individual patients and this likely relates to the sites of metastatic disease. The biology of the tumor and its progression may be different in patients with visceral versus nonvisceral disease. It is unclear if the sites of metastasis are the cause or result of the varied biologic behavior in individual patients.

SINGLE CHEMOTHERAPY AGENTS

The response rate of patients with metastatic melanoma to single chemotherapeutic agents is low. DTIC is the most active drug and results in response rates of 15–25%.[8,9] Patients with skin, subcutaneous tissue or lymph node metastases respond most frequently while those with liver and brain metastases rarely respond. Complete responses rarely occur and the usual duration of partial responses is only 5–6 months. DTIC toxicities may be substantial and include nausea, vomiting, moderate myelosuppression, flu-like syndrome, and rarely fulminant hepatic venoocclusive disease.

Other chemotherapeutic drugs with activity in metastatic melanoma include: nitrosoureas such as BCNU (carmustine), CCNU and methyl CCNU;[10] vinca alkaloids (vinblastine, vincristine);[11,12] and cisplatin.[13,14] The response rates with these drugs vary from 10–20% and are usually partial and of short duration.

Recently, several new strategies for using cisplatin in patients with metastatic melanoma have been studied. Glover et al initially reported a 70% overall response rate using high dose (150 mg/m^2) cisplatin combined with WR-2721.[15] WR-2721 is a phosphorothioic acid derivative that decreases cisplatin normal tissue toxicity in preclinical models. More recent followup studies using these agents were less promising. Avril et al reported a 35% response rate (duration 2 to 15 weeks) in 20 patients treated with cisplatin 120 mg/m^2 and WR-2721.[16] Buzaid et al saw no responses in six evaluable patients using split dose (day 1, 8) cisplatin 100 mg/m^2 combined with WR-2721.[17]

Standard single agent chemotherapy cannot be routinely recommended for patients with metastatic melanoma. These patients should be considered for participation on clinical trials of new treatment approaches or treated with combination therapy.

NEW CHEMOTHERAPY AGENTS

The search for new chemotherapy drugs to treat patients with metastatic melanoma remains an active area of investigation. Over the past 20–25 years several new agents have shown initial promise but were later discarded after study in larger groups of patients confirmed response rates no better than those seen with single agent DTIC. The following discussion will focus on new agents tested in the past few years.

Fotemustine (diethyl-1-[3-2 chloro-ethyl]-3-nitroso-ureido ethyl phosphonate) is a novel nitrosourea that recently entered phase II clinical trials in patients with metastatic melanoma. Schallreuter et al reported a 47% overall response rate in 19 patients [2 – complete responses (CR), 7 – partial responses (PR)].[18] Toxicity was relatively mild and included thrombocytopenia, leukopenia, nausea and vomiting. Jacquillat et al treated 153 evaluable metastatic melanoma patients including those with cerebral metastases.[19] The overall response rate to fotemustine was 24% (2% – CR, 22% – PR) and the primary toxicity was hematologic. The median duration of response was 22 weeks (range 7–80 weeks). Responses were seen in cerebral (25%), visceral (19%), and non-visceral (31.8%) sites. The overall response rate in previously untreated patients was 31%. Fotemustine is worthy of further study in metastatic melanoma because of the overall promising response rates compared to other single agents, the activity in cerebral and other visceral metastases and tolerable toxicity.

Taxol is a natural product antitumor agent isolated from the bark of the western yew tree (*Taxus brevifolia*). It blocks cell replication via stabilization of cytoplasmic microtubules.[20] Taxol has shown activity in patients with breast and ovarian cancer.[21] Einzig et al treated 34 patients with metastatic melanoma using taxol 250 mg/m^2 as a 24 hour infusion with a 21 day treatment cycle.[22] Three complete responses and one partial response were observed for an overall

response rate of 14% in 28 evaluable patients who had not previously received chemotherapy. Toxicities included acute hypersensitivity reactions (11%), neutropenia (68%) and peripheral neuropathy (59%).

A major obstacle to further clinical studies of taxol is the tedious purification process and resultant limited drug supply. Taxotere is a semisynthetic analog of taxol. It is more readily available than taxol because it can be synthesized in vitro using a precursor obtained from a renewable resource (the needles of *Taxus baccata*). In preclinical studies taxotere was active against mouse B16 melanoma and shows greater tumor inhibition than taxol in this model.[23] Further study of taxol and/ or taxotere alone or in combination with other agents in patients with metastatic melanoma is warranted.

Piritrexim is a new lipid soluble dihydrofolate reductase (DHFR) inhibitor. Piritrexim differs from the classical DHFR inhibitor, methotrexate in that it gains more rapid and efficient cellular entry.[24] Feun et al conducted a phase II trial of piritrexim in 31 patients with metastatic melanoma.[25] Two complete responses and five partial responses were observed for an overall response rate of 23%. The responses occurred primarily in soft tissue and lung. Piritrexim was relatively well tolerated and the most consistent toxicity was myelosuppression. Piritrexim appears more active than methotrexate in metastatic melanoma and is worthy of further study.

Daily oral etoposide[26] and fludarabine[27] have also been studied in phase II trials in patients with metastatic melanoma. No responses were seen in 27 patients treated with fludarabine and 17 patients treated with oral etoposide. Both agents should be considered inactive.

COMBINATION CHEMOTHERAPY

The use of combination chemotherapy in metastatic melanoma was long considered of minimal benefit because the response rate and patient survival were not substantially different than those seen with single agent DTIC. However, in recent

mg orally twice daily).[28] They initially treated 20 patients with metastatic melanoma and 11 (55%) achieved objective response (4 – CR, 7 – PR). In a followup study McClay et al treated 20 patients with metastatic melanoma using the same combination regimen and observed a 50% response rate (all partial remissions).[29] The median duration of response in these studies was 10 months and >7 months, respectively. Patients relapsing after

Table 1. Combination Chemotherapy for Metastatic Melanoma

Reference	Regimen	No. Pts	%CR	%PR	Over-all Response (%)
McClay et al, 1992	DTIC, CDDP, BCNU, Tam	45	11	40	51
Cocconi et al, 1990	DTIC, Tam	60	7	22	29
Ferri et al, 1992	DTIC, CBDCA, Tam	22	5	18	23
Buzaid et al, 1991	DTIC, CDDP, Tam	23	9	4	13
Legha et al, 1989	DTIC, CDDP, VBL	50	4	36	40
Luger et al, 1990	DTIC, CDDP	28	25	4	29
Murren et al, 1991	DTIC, CDDP	22	18	14	32
Steffens et al, 1991	DTIC, CDDP	30	0	17	17
Avril et al, 1990	DTIC, fotemustine	63	14	19	33

Abbreviations: DTIC - dacarbazine, CDDP - cisplatin, BCNU - carmustine, Tam - tamoxifen, VBL - vinblastine, CBDCA - carboplatin, CR - complete remission, PR - partial remission

years the use of combination chemo-hormonal therapy and chemoimmunotherapy (discussed in the following section) resulted in improved response rates. (Table 1)

In 1984 Del Prete et al reported a combination chemotherapy regimen using DTIC (220 mg/m^2 days 1–3 every three weeks), cisplatin (25 mg/m^2 days 1–3 every three weeks), BCNU (150 mg/m^2 day 1 every six weeks) and tamoxifen (10

treatment with this regimen commonly developed CNS metastases and there was a high incidence of deep venus thrombosis and the pulmonary embolism.

In an attempt to reduce the incidence of thrombotic events the tamoxifen was dropped from the regimen and an additional 20 patients were treated by McClay et al.[30] Without the tamoxifen no patients developed deep venous thrombosis or pulmonary embolism, but the overall response rate decreased to 10% (1 – CR, 1 – PR). When tamoxifen was re-incorporated into the regimen the response increased to 52% in a third group of 25 additional patients.[31] Thus, it was concluded the tamoxifen was an important component of this regimen.

The mechanism of interaction of tamoxifen with the cytotoxic drugs in this regimen is under investigation but currently unknown. Recently, McClay et al treated 21 melanoma patients (15 evaluable) with single agent cisplatin. Patients who progressed were then treated with combination cisplatin and tamoxifen. Four patients demonstrated partial remission to the combination after failing single agent cisplatin.[32] Additional data shows cisplatin and tamoxifen are synergistic in vitro against melanoma cell lines but the biochemical mechanism remains unclear.[32]

In a study by Cocconi et al patients were randomized to receive DTIC alone (52 patients) or DTIC plus tamoxifen (60 patients).[33] The two treatment arms contained similar numbers of patients with visceral and non-visceral disease. DTIC alone resulted in a 12% overall response rate whereas DTIC plus tamoxifen resulted in a 28% response rate (p = 0.03). In addition, median survival duration was increased in patients receiving the combination (48 versus 29 weeks, p = 0.07). A randomized comparison of carboplatin and DTIC versus carboplatin, DTIC and tamoxifen is underway[34] but the results to date are inconclusive.

Buzaid et al used a high dose loading scheme for tamoxifen (100 mg twice daily for seven days followed by 10 mg twice daily) in combination with DTIC and high dose cisplatin (50 mg/m² days 1–3).[37]

Their results were disappointing in that of 23 evaluable patients only three developed objective responses (13%).

Legha et al treated 50 patients with a non-tamoxifen containing combination chemotherapy regimen employing cisplatin, vinblastine and DTIC.[35] They observed an overall 40% response rate (4% CR). The median response duration was 9 months. The regimen was associated with significant toxicity including nausea, vomiting, diarrhea and alopecia.

Other investigators used escalating cisplatin doses in combination with DTIC.[36-38] (Table 1) The overall response rates varied from 17% to 32%. The toxicity of these regimens was occasionally severe and included nausea, vomiting, neuropathy, ototoxicity, potassium and magnesium depletion and myelosuppression.[37,38] Due to the toxicity and modest response rates this treatment approach is not recommended.

Avril et al treated 63 patients (32% had received prior cytotoxic chemotherapy) with DTIC combined with a new nitrosourea, fotemustine.[39] The overall response rate was 33% (9 – CR, 12 – PR). Responses also occurred in cerebral (29%) and visceral (23%) sites. Because this regimen appears active in previously treated patients and in those with cerebral and/or visceral metastases it is worthy of further study.

In summary, it is now clear that combination chemotherapy regimens employing DTIC, cisplatin, BCNU and tamoxifen result in increased response rates relative to treatment with DTIC alone. There is also evidence supporting synergy between cisplatin and tamoxifen and DTIC and tamoxifen. However, the majority of the responses observed are partial and a consistent and significant increase in patient survival has not been shown. In addition, many patients who relapse develop CNS metastases and thus have an extremely poor prognosis. New treatment approaches include frequent observation for CNS metastases with head CT scans, prophylactic brain radiotherapy, use of drugs with activity for CNS disease such as fotemustine and use of combination chemoimmunotherapy (discussed in the next section).

Richards et al recently reported that patients with metastatic melanoma who failed treatment with interleukin-2 can respond to the DTIC, cisplatin, BCNU, tamoxifen regimen.[40] In 20 patients they observed 11 partial responses (55%). These results indicate that these chemotherapy drugs and interleukin-2 are non-cross resistant and provide further rationale for combination chemoimmunotherapy regimens.

COMBINATION CHEMOIMMUNOTHERAPY

Immunotherapeutic approaches for treatment of metastatic melanoma (discussed by Hersh et al in this volume) have met with modest success. The most actively studied biologic agents are interleukin-2 (IL-2) and Interferon—α (IFN—α). Because immunotherapy and chemotherapy likely have different mechanisms of antitumor action (indirect immunomodulation versus direct cytotoxicity) it is reasonable to consider combination chemoimmunotherapy regimens. However, the combination may also result in synergistic or additive toxicity and thus limit patient tolerance.

CHEMOTHERAPY PLUS INTERFERON—α

IFN—α has modest activity as a single agent in the treatment of metastatic melanoma. In many series of patients employing varied doses, schedules and routes of administration the overall response rate ranges from 3–29%.[41] The antitumor activity of IFN is felt to be primarily related to its antiproliferative effects rather than immunomodulatory effects.[42] Garbe et al reported in vitro evidence for synergy of IFN with cisplatin, vindesine and BCNU.[42]

In phase II trials of recombinant Interferon—α2a (rIFN—α2a) combined with DTIC overall response rates varied from 23–35%.[43-45] (Table 2) It can be concluded from the phase II trials that this combination is tolerable and the response rate is perhaps slightly better than that of DTIC alone.

Three randomized clinical trials have been performed comparing DTIC versus DTIC plus rIFN—α. (Table 2) Kirkwood et al reported preliminary results of a three arm randomized clinical trial: DTIC (250 mg/m^2/day for five days every three weeks) versus IFN—α2b (30 x 10^6 U/day for five days every week for three weeks, then 10 x 10^6 U/m^2 SC three times per week) versus the combination.[46] The results are presented in Table 2 and show no difference between the response rates for DTIC alone and DTIC plus rIFN—α2b. The response to rIFN—α2b alone was lower than most previously reported studies.

Falkson et al randomly assigned 61 patients to receive either DTIC (200 mg/m^2 IV daily for 5 days, repeated every 28 days) versus DTIC plus rIFN—α2b (15 x 10^6 U/m^2 IV daily for five days per week

Table 2. Chemotherapy Plus Interferon-α

Reference	Regimen	No. Pts.	%CR	%PR	Over-all Response (%)
Bajetta et al, 1990	DTIC, rIFN−α2a	75	8	17	25
Mulder et al, 1990	DTIC, rIFN−α2a	31	10	26	35
Hersey et al, 1991	DTIC, rIFN−α2a	76	9	17	26
Hersey et al, 1991	DTIC, rIFN−α2a	30	7	17	23
Kirkwood et al, 1990	DTIC	24	NA	NA	20
	versus				
	rIFN−α2b	23	NA	NA	4
	versus				
	DTIC, rIFN−α2b	21	NA	NA	19
Falkson et al, 1991	DTIC	31	6	13	20
	versus				
	DTIC, rIFN−α2b	30	40	13	53
Sertoli et al, 1992	DTIC	67	4	12	16
	versus				
	DTIC, rIFN−α2a(HD)	62	6	21	27
	versus				
	DTIC, rIFN−α2a(LD)	74	7	18	25
Gröhn et al, 1992	DTIC, nimustine, rIFN−α2b	52	17	6	23
Morton et al, 1991	BCNU, rIFN−α2a	30	3	3	7

Abbreviations: DTIC - dacarbazine, rIFN - recombinant interferon, BCNU - carmustine, CR - complete response, PR - partial response, HD - high dose, LD - low dose, NA - not available

for three weeks, then 10×10^6 U/m^2 SC three times per week).[47] The results in Table 2 show a significantly increased response rate for the combination (53% versus 20%, p = 0.007). Median survival time was 9.6 months for DTIC alone and 17.6 months for DTIC plus rIFN−α2b (p < 0.01). Hematologic toxicity, neurologic toxicity and flu-like symptoms were more severe in patients receiving the combin-ation. It was concluded that the combination of DTIC and rIFN−α2b is significantly better than DTIC alone and further confirmatory randomized trials are in progress.

Sertoli et al recently reported in abstract form a randomized trial of DTIC (800 mg/m^2 every 21 days) versus DTIC plus rIFN−α2a (9 x 10^6 U IM daily for six months) versus DTIC plus lower dose rIFN−α2a (3 x 10^6 U IM three times weekly).[48] As shown in Table 2 there was no substantial difference in response rate among the three treatment arms. However, duration of complete or partial response was greater on the DTIC plus IFN−α2a arms (2.6 versus 6.6 and 9 months, respectively).

The reason for different results among the three randomized clinical trials of

DTIC plus IFN−α are not readily apparent. Both the studies by Kirkwood et al and Falkson et al employed a high dose loading scheme for interferon (30 x 10^6 U/day SC for five days every three weeks versus 15 x 10^6 U/m^2 IV daily for five days per week for three weeks, respectively). The total IFN dose in these two trials is similar but the trial by Falkson administered the interferon IV. Further study is needed to clarify this issue.

Two additional studies combining rIFN−α with DTIC and nimustine (a nitrosourea)[49] and BCNU[50] are shown in Table 2. The overall response rates are not different than previously reported combinations.

for patients with metastatic melanoma by Rosenberg et al.[51] A summary of subsequent trials of rIL-2 in melanoma show an overall response rate of approximately 20% with 10% of patients developing complete responses.[52] A number of combination chemotherapy regimens have been combined with rIL-2 and are summarized in Table 3.

Demchak et al treated 27 patients with cisplatin (150 mg/m^2 plus WR-2721 day 1 only or 50 mg/m^2 days 1,2,3 without WR-2721) plus rIL-2 (600,000 IU/kg IV q eight hours days 1-5 and 15-19).[53] The overall response rate was 37% with 11% complete responses. The toxicity of this regimen was typical of high dose rIL-2 and included nephrotoxicity, pulmonary

---

Table 3. Chemotherapy Plus Interleukin-2

Reference	Regimen	No. Pts.	%CR	%PR	Over-all Response (%)
Demchak et al, 1991	CDDP, rIL-2	27	11	26	37
Flaherty et al, 1990	DTIC, rIL-2	32	3	19	22
Flaherty et al, 1992	DTIC, CDDP	7	0	57	57
	versus				
	DTIC, CDDP, rIL-2	8	0	63	63
Mitchell, 1989	CPA, IL-2	39	5	21	26
Verdi et al, 1992	CPA, IL-2	23	0	4	4

Abbreviations: CDDP - cisplatin, rIL-2 - recombinant interleukin-2, DTIC - dacarbazine, CPA - cyclophosphamide

---

CHEMOTHERAPY PLUS INTERLEUKIN-2

Recombination interleukin-2 (rIL-2) combined with lymphokine activated killer (LAK) cells was first used as therapy

toxicity, weight gain, cardiac toxicity, nausea and vomiting, but there were no treatment related deaths. It was concluded that this regimen was active but toxic.

Flaherty et al performed a combination chemoimmunotherapy trial employing DTIC plus rIL-2.[54] The dose of rIL-2 was escalated from 12 to 30 x 10[6] IU/m². The overall response rate (22%) was not substantially better than previous reports with DTIC alone. The same group recently reported preliminary results of a randomized trial comparing DTIC and cisplatin versus DTIC, cisplatin and rIL-2.[55] (Table 3) The response rate in both treatment arms was greater than 50%. However, all responses were partial and only small numbers of patients have been treated thus far.

A different approach using rIL-2 combined with chemotherapy drugs was reported by Mitchell et al.[56] Low dose cyclophosphamide (350 mg/m²) preceded low dose rIL-2 (21.6 x 10[6] IU/m²/day five days per week for two weeks). The cyclophosphamide was given primarily for its immunomodulatory effects (decrease T-suppressor cells and humoral suppressor factors) rather than its direct cytotoxic effects. An update of this study showed a 26% overall response rate in 39 patients.[57] This regimen had tolerable toxicity and could be delivered in an outpatient setting. A similar regimen of rIL-2 combined with cyclophosphamide was recently employed by Verdi et al.[58] This group treated 23 patients with malignant melanoma and saw only one partial remission (overall response rate 4%).

CHEMOTHERAPY PLUS INTERFERON-α AND INTERLEUKIN-2

The next logical step in the progression of chemoimmunotherapy studies for melanoma was to give combination chemotherapy plus both rIL-2 and rIFN-α. Three such studies were recently reported in preliminary form. (Table 4)

Khayat et al used a regimen of cisplatin (100 mg/m² day 1), rIL-2 (18 x 10[6] IU/m²/day by 24 hour IV infusion, days 3-6 and 17-21) and simultaneous rIFN-α (9 x 10[6] units SC three times weekly).[59] They treated 20 patients (18 previously treated with chemotherapy and 10 previously treated with IFN) and observed an overall response rate of 60% (20% - CR, 40% - PR). The toxicity of this regimen was substantial. Fourteen patients developed grade III hypotension and required low doses of dopamine. Other toxicity included renal, hematologic, fever, chills, nausea, vomiting and diarrhea.

Legha et al extended their previous experience with the DTIC, cisplatin, vinblastine regimen and added rIL-2 (3 x 10[6] U/m²/day administered in the hospital

Table 4. Chemotherapy Plus Interferon-α and Interleukin-2

Reference	Regimen	No. Pts.	%CR	%PR	Over-all Response (%)
Khyat et al, 1992	CDDP, rIL-2, rIFN-α	20	20	40	60
Legha et al, 1992	DTIC, CDDP, VBL, rIL-2, rIFN-α	30	20	37	56
Richards et al, 1992	DTIC, CDDP, BCNU, rIL-2, rIFN-α	74	15	40	55

Abbreviations: CDDP - cisplatin, rIL-2 - recombinant IL-2, rIFN-α - recombinant interferon-α DTIC - dacarbazine, BCNU - carmustine, VBL - vinblastine

by continuous IV infusion for 96 hours) and rIFN–α (5 x 10^6 U/m^2 for five days weekly) alternating with the chemotherapy regimen.[60] An overall response rate of 56% was observed. (Table 4) Significant multi-system toxicity was again observed. Nineteen patients developed neutropenic sepsis and 14 required platelet transfusion. However, there were no treatment-related deaths.

Richards et al recently reported the extension of their previous experience with the DTIC, cisplatin, BCNU and tamoxifen regimen combined with rIL-2 (1.5 x 10^6 U/m^2 q eight hours days 4–8 and 17–21) plus rIFN–α2a (6 x 10^6 U/m^2 SC days 4–8 and 17–21).[61] Fifty-five percent of 74 patients developed objective response. The median time to development of progressive disease was 9.1 months and the median survival was 14 months.

In summary, the most active combination chemoimmunotherapy regimens for metastatic melanoma reported thus far use both rIL-2 and rIFN–α combined with chemotherapy as reported in Table 4. The numbers of patients treated with these regimens and the consistent response rate greater than 50% are encouraging. However, severe toxicity is associated with this treatment approach and it is likely that the patients entered on these studies were highly selected for good performance status and ability to tolerate potentially severe toxicity. Further study of these regimens is warranted.

HIGH DOSE CHEMOTHERAPY WITH BONE MARROW TRANSPLANTATION

An aggressive approach to treatment of refractory solid tumors uses high dose chemotherapy with autologous bone marrow transplantation (ABMT) as rescue for the associated severe myelosuppression. This approach has met with success and is now commonly employed in patients with breast cancer, non-Hodgkin's lymphoma and Hodgkin's disease. A number of groups have also investigated this approach in patients with metastatic melanoma. (Table 5)

Tchekmedyian et al treated 18 patients with high dose BCNU, vincristine and melphalan but did not administer ABMT.[62] The overall response rate was low (22%) and the median response duration was only five months. In addition, 26% of patients died after the first course of BCNU before achieving bone marrow recovery. This treatment regimen cannot be recommended.

Shea et al used a regimen of high dose cyclophosphamide, cisplatin, BCNU plus ABMT in 19 patients with metastatic melanoma.[63] The overall response rate was excellent (58%) but most responses were partial (53%) and the response duration was short (4.7 months).

Thatcher et al used three high dose chemotherapy plus ABMT regimens: high dose DTIC and melphalan, lower dose DTIC and melphalan, and DTIC plus ifosfamide.[64] The overall response rate across all regimens was 49% with a median response duration of 4.5 months. However, with the high dose DTIC and melphalan regimen the overall response rate was 81% (25% complete response). Hematologic and gastrointestinal toxicity were severe and one patient treated with high dose DTIC and melphalan died of septicemia.

Wolff et al evaluated escalating doses of thiotepa and ABMT.[65] The response

Table 5. High Dose Chemotherapy With or Without Autologous Bone Marrow Transplantation

Reference	Regimen	No. Pts.	%CR	%PR	Over-all Response (%)	Median Response Duration (mos)
Tchekmedyian et al, 1986	BCNU, VCR/MEL	18	0	22	22	5
Shea et al, 1988	CPA, CDDP, BCNU plus ABMT	19	5	53	58	4.7
Thatcher et al, 1989	DTIC, MEL or IFO plus ABMT	37	14	35	49	4.5
Wolff et al, 1989	Thiotepa plus ABMT	55	7	46	53	3
Lakhani et al, 1990	VDN or MEL or BCNU or BLEO, VCR, DTIC, CCNU plus ABMT	154	5	10	15	3
Meisenberg et al, 1992	CPA, CDDP, BCNU plus ABMT	15	40	27	67	2.5

Abbreviations: BCNU - carmustine, VCR - vincristine, MEL - melphalan, CPA - cyclophosphamide, CDDP - cisplatin, ABMT - autologous bone marrow transplantation, DTIC - dacarbazine, IFO - ifosfamide, VDN - vindesine, BLEO - bleomycin, CCNU - lomustine

rate in 55 evaluable patients was 53% overall with the majority being partial responses. The median response duration was only three months but 10% of the responses lasted more than one year.

Lakhani et al reported a large series (154 evaluable patients) treated with four different high dose chemotherapy regimens and ABMT: high dose vindesine, high dose melphalan, high dose BCNU or the BOLD regimen (bleomycin, vincristine, CCNU, DTIC).[66] The response rate across all regimens was 15% with a three month median response duration.

Among the four regimens the best response rate was observed in the high dose BCNU treated patients (44% CR plus PR). However, there was no difference in overall survival among the four regimens.

Recently, Meisenberg et al treated 15 melanoma patients with relapse after surgery for stage II melanoma.[67] The overall response rate was 67% (40% – CR, 27% – PR) but again the response duration was only 2.5 months.

In summary, the use of high dose chemotherapy and ABMT for patients with malignant melanoma must be considered highly experimental. This treatment approach generally results in response rates of about 50%. However, the treatment is expensive, extremely toxic and carries a definite risk of early mortality associated with the treatment. The duration of responses are uniformly short (3–5 months).

CONCLUSIONS AND FUTURE PROSPECTS

The chance of long term benefit for patients with metastatic melanoma treated with chemotherapy, chemoimmunotherapy or any other modality remains small. However, there is reason for cautious optimism and continued basic and clinical research to develop new drugs and new drug combinations with activity in this disease.

Among the recently studied new drugs for metastatic melanoma, the most promising are taxol, fotemustine and piritrexim. The activity of these drugs as single agents is sufficient to warrant incorporation into combination chemotherapy or chemoimmunotherapy regimens. However, the search for drugs with greater anti-tumor activity and specificity for melanoma should continue.

The combination chemotherapy regimen using DTIC, CDDP, BCNU and tamoxifen originally reported by Del Prete et al and extensively studied by McClay et al and the DTIC, CDDP vinblastine regimen reported by Legha et al are active in 40 to 50% of patients with metastatic melanoma. However, there are a number of problems with these regimens: most responses are partial, the survival and natural history of metastatic melanoma patients is not consistently altered, and

patients commonly relapse within the CNS. Evidence supporting the importance of tamoxifen in the first regimen is accumulating, but the exact mechanism of the interaction remains unknown and should be the focus of continued basic studies. Future combination chemotherapy clinical trials should incorporate new active drugs as they are identified, especially those with CNS activity such as fotemustine.

The combination chemoimmunotherapy regimens employing IL-2 and IFN–α are active in 50–60% of patients with metastatic melanoma. However, the clinical trials reported thus far have treated relatively few patients that were highly selected. In addition, it is not clear if survival is improved by this treatment approach and it is potentially very toxic. Further study of this approach in controlled clinical trials and evaluation of other cytokines such as interleukin-4 and IFN-γ in combination with chemotherapy drugs is warranted.

High dose chemotherapy plus ABMT cannot be recommended as standard therapy for patients with metastatic melanoma due to the severe toxicity, short duration of response and expense. However, novel approaches employing hematopoietic growth factors to lessen the duration of bone marrow aplasia and immunotherapeutic approaches with cytokines as maintenance therapy after remission induction are worthy of study in clinical trials.

In the past 10 years the use of chemotherapy for metastatic melanoma has progressed from the dismal prospect of a 10–15% chance of response with single agent DTIC and no added benefit with combination therapy to the present where 40–60% of patients can reasonably be expected to respond with aggressive therapy. However, it can be argued that a major impact on this disease has not occurred because survival is not consistently improved with today's treatment approaches. Thus, all eligible patients with metastatic melanoma should be offered participation on well designed clinical trials that will hopefully continue the progress made in the last 10 years.

References

1. McNeer G, Das Gupta TK. Prognosis in malignant melanoma. Surgery 1964; 56:512.

2. Ketcham AS, Balch CM. Classification and staging systems In: Balch CM and Milton GW, eds. Cutaneous Melanoma: Clinical Management and Treatment Results Worldwide. Philadelphia: J.B. Lippincott, 1985:55

3. Balch CM, Soong SJ, Murad TM et al. A multifactorial analysis of melanoma: IV. Prognostic factors in 200 melanoma patients with distant metastases. J Clin Oncol 1983; 1:126.

4. Devesa SS, Silverman DT, Young JLJ. Cancer incidence and mortality trends among whites in the United States. J Natl Cancer Inst 1987; 79:701-70.

5. Boring CC, Squires TS, Tong T. Cancer Statistics 1991. Ca-A Cancer J Clinicians 1991; 41:19-36.

6. Balch CM, Soong SJ, Shaw HM. An analysis of prognostic factors in 4000 patients with cutaneous melanoma. In: Balch CM and Milton GW, eds. Cutaneous Melanoma: Clinical Management and Treatment Results Worldwide. Philadelphia: J.B. Lippincott, 1985:321.

7. Joensuu H. Association between chemotherapy response and rate of disease progression in disseminated melanoma. Br J Cancer 1991; 63:154-6.

8. Pritchard KI, Quirt IC, Cowan DH et al.

DTIC therapy in metastatic malignant melanoma: a simplified dose schedule. Cancer Treat Rep 1980; 64:1123-6.

9. Comis RL, Carter SK. Integration of chemotherapy into combined modality therapy of solid tumors: Malignant melanoma. Cancer Treat Rev 1974; 1:285-304.

10. Luce JK. Chemotherapy of malignant melanoma. Cancer 1972; 30:1604-15.

11. Falkson G, Van Dyk JJ, Verwoerd HF. The chemotherapy of malignant melanoma. S Afr Med J 1968; 42:89-90.

12. Nathanson L, Wittenberg BK. Pilot study of vinblastine and bleomycin combinations in the treatment of metastatic melanoma. Cancer Treat Rep 1980; 64:133-7.

13. Al-Sarraf M, Fletcher W, Oishi N et al. Cisplatin hydration with and without mannitol diuresis in refractory disseminated malignant melanoma: A Southwest Oncology Group Study. Cancer Treat Rep 1982; 66:31-5.

14. Mechl Z, Krejci P. Cis-diaminedichloroplatinum in the treatment of disseminated malignant melanoma. Neoplasma 1983; 30:371-7.

15. Glover D, Grabelsky S, Weiler C et al. Toxicity and antitumor activity of WR-2721 and cisplatin (DDP) 150 mg/m². Proc ASCO 1989; 8:65

16. Avril MF, Ortoli JC, Fortier-Beaulieu M et al. High dose cisplatin and WR 2721 in metastatic melanoma. Proc ASCO 1992; 11:344.

17. Buzaid AC, Murren JR, Durivage HJ. High-dose cisplatin with dacarbazine and tamoxifen in the treatment of metastatic melanoma. Cancer 1991; 68:1238-41.

18. Schallreuter KU, Wenzel E, Brassow FW et al. Positive phase-II study in the treatment of advanced malignant melanoma with fotemustine. Cancer Chemother Pharmacol 1991; 29:85-7.

19. Jacquillat C, Khayat D, Banzet P et al. Final report of the French multicenter phase II study of the nitrosourea fotemustine in 153 evaluable patients with disseminated malignant melanoma

including patients with cerebral metastases. Cancer 1990; 66:1873-8.

20. Schiff PB, Horwitz SB. Taxol stabilizes microtubules in mouse fibroblast cells. Proc Natl Acad Sci 1980; 77:1561-5.

21. Slichenmyer WJ., Vonhoff DD. Taxol – A new and effective anti-cancer drug. Anti-Cancer Drugs 1991; 2:519-30.

22. Einzig AI, Hochster H, Wiernik PH et al. A Phase II study of taxol in patients with malignant melanoma. Inv New Drugs 1991; 9:59-64.

23. Bissery MC, Guenard D, Guerittevoegelein F et al. Experimental antitumor activity of taxotere (RP-56976, NSC-628503), a taxol analogue. Cancer Res 1991; 51:4845-52.

24. Duch DS, Edelstein MP, Bowers SW. Biochemical and chemotherapeutic studies in 2,4-diamino-6 (2,5-dimethoxybenzyl)-5methyl pyrido (2,3d) pyrimidine (BW 30lu). A novel lipid-soluble inhibitor of dihydrofolate reductase. Cancer Res 1982; 42:3987-94.

25. Feun LG, Gonzalez R, Savaraj N.et al. Phase-II trial of piritrexim in metastatic melanoma using intermittent, low-dose administration. J Clin Oncol 1991; 9:464-7.

26. Whittaker T, Schultz S, Rynard S. Phase II study of daily oral VP-16 in metastatic melanoma: a Hoosier Oncology Group (HOG) study. Proc ASCO 1992; 11:348.

27. Kish JA, Kopecky K, Samson MK et al. Evaluation of fludarabine phosphate in malignant melanoma. Inv New Drugs 1991; 9:105-8.

28. Del Prete SA, Maurer LH, O'Donnell J et al. Combination chemotherapy with cisplatin, carmustine, dacarbazine, and tamoxifen in metastatic melanoma. Cancer Treat Rep 1984; 68:1403-5.

29. McClay EF, Mastrangelo MJ, Bellet RE, Berd D. Combination chemotherapy and hormonal therapy in the treatment of malignant melanoma. Cancer Treat Rep 1987; 71:465-9.

30. McClay EF, Mastrangelo MJ, Sprandio JD et al. The importance of tamoxifen to a cisplatin-containing regimen in the treatment of metastatic melanoma. Cancer 1989; 63:1292-5.

31. McClay EF, Mastrangelo MJ, Berd D, Bellet RE. Effective combination chemohormonal therapy for malignant melanoma: experience with three consecutive trials. Int J Cancer 1992; 50:553-6.

32. McClay EF, Albright K, Jones J et al. Modulation of cisplatin (DDP) resistance by tamoxifen (TAM) in human malignant melanoma. Proc ASCO 1992; 11:343.

33. Cocconi G, Bella M, Calabresi F et al. DTIC vs DTIC plus tamoxifen in metastatic malignant melanoma. Proc ASCO 1990; 9:278.

34. Ferri W, Kirkwood JM, Vlock D et al. Phase II trial of carboplatin and dacarbazine plus tamoxifen in metastatic melanoma. Proc ASCO 1992; 11:349

35. Legha SS, Ring S, Papadopoulos N et al. A prospective evaluation of a triple-drug regimen containing cisplatin, vinblastine and dacarbazine (CVD) for metastatic melanoma. Cancer 1989; 64: 2024-9.

36. Murren JR, Derosa W, Durivage HJ et al. High-dose cisplatin plus dacarbazine in the treatment of metastatic melanoma. Cancer 1991; 67:1514-17.

37. Luger SM, Kirkwood JM, Ernstoff MS, Vlock DR. High-dose cisplatin and dacarbazine in the treatment of metastatic melanoma. J Natl Cancer Inst 1990; 82:1934-7.

38. Steffens TA, Bajorin DF, Chapman PB et al. A phase II trial of high-dose cisplatin and dacarbazine - lack of efficacy of high-dose, cisplatin-based therapy for metastatic melanoma. Cancer 1991; 68:1230-7.

39. Avril MF, Bonneterre J, Delaunay M et al. Combination chemotherapy of dacarbazine and fotemustine in disseminated malignant melanoma. Cancer Chemother Pharmacol 1990; 27:81-4.

40. Richards JM, Gilewski TA, Ramming K et al. Effective chemotherapy for melanoma after treatment with interleukin-2. Cancer 1992; 69:427-9.

41. McClay EF, Mastrangelo MJ. Systemic chemotherapy for metastatic

melanoma. Semin Oncol 1988; 15:569-77.

42. Garbe C, Kreuser ED, Zouboulis CC et al. Combined treatment of metastatic melanoma with interferons and cytotoxic drugs. Semin Oncol 1992; 19:63-9.

43. Mulder NH, Willemse PHB, Koops HS et al. Dacarbazine (DTIC) and human recombinant interferon alpha-2a (Roferon) in the treatment of disseminated malignant melanoma. Br J Cancer 1990; 62:1006-7.

44. Bajetta E, Negretti E, Giannotti B et al. Phase II study of interferon α-2a and dacarbazine in advanced melanoma. Am J Clin Oncol 1990; 13:405-9.

45. Hersey P, Mcleod GRC, Thomson DB. Treatment of advanced malignant melanoma with recombinant Interferon-alfa-2a in combination with DTIC - long-term follow-up of two phase-II studies. Br J Haematol 1991; 79:60-6.

46. Kirkwood JM, Giuliano EA, Gams R et al. Interferon α-2a and dacarbazine in melanoma. J Natl Cancer Inst 1990; 82:1062-3.

47. Falkson CI, Falkson G, Falkson HC. Improved results with the addition of interferon alfa-2b to Dacarbazine in the treatment of patients with metastatic malignant melanoma. J Clin Oncol 1991; 9:1403-8.

48. Sertoli MR, Queirolo P, Bajetta E et al. Dacarbazine (DTIC) with or without recombinant interferon alpha-2a at different dosages in the treatment of stage IV melanoma patients. Proc ASCO 1992; 11:345.

49. Gröhn P, Kumpulainen E, Nuortio L et al. A phase-II study of metastatic melanoma treated with a combination of Interferon-alfa-2b, dacarbazine and nimustine. Eur J Cancer 1992; 28:441-3.

50. Morton RF, Creagan ET, Schaid DJ.et al. Phase II trial of recombinant leukocyte A interferon (IFN−α2A) plus 1,3-Bis(2-Chloroethyl)-1-nitrosourea (BCNU) and the combination cimetidine with BCNU in patients with disseminated

malignant melanoma. Am J Clin Oncol 1991; 14:152-5.

51. Rosenberg SA, Lotze MT, Muul,LM. Observations on the systemic administration of autologous lymphokine-activated killer cells and recombinant interleukin-2 to patients with metastatic cancer. N Engl J Med 1985; 313:1485-92, 1985.

52. Sznol M, Dutcher JP, Atkins MB et al. Review of interleukin-2 alone and interleukin-2/LAK clinical trials in metastatic malignant melanoma. Cancer Treat Rev 1989; 16:29-38.

53. Demchak PA, Mier JW, Robert NJ et al. Interleukin-2 and high-dose cisplatin in patients with metastatic melanoma - a pilot study. J Clin Oncol 1991; 9:1821-30.

54. Flaherty LE, Redman BG, Chabot GG et al. A phase I-II study of dacarbazine in combination with outpatient interleukin-2 in metastatic malignant melanoma. Cancer 1990; 65:2471-7.

55. Flaherty L, Redman B, Martino S et al. High dose dacarbazine (DTIC) and cisplatin alone and combined with outpatient interleukin-2 (IL-2) in metastatic malignant melanoma. Proc ASCO 1992; 11:350.

56. Mitchell MS. Chemotherapy in combination with biomodulation - a five-year experience with cyclophosphamide and interleukin-2. Semin Oncol 1992; 19: 80-7.

57. Mitchell MS, Kempf RA, Harel W et al. Low-dose cyclophosphamide and low-dose interleukin-2 for malignant melanoma. Bull NY Acad Med 1989; 65:128-44.

58. Verdi CJ, Taylor CW, Croghan MK et al. Phase-I study of low-dose cyclophosphamide and recombinant interleukin-2 for the treatment of advanced cancer. J Immunother 1992; 11:286-91.

59. Khayat D, Borel CH, Antoine E et al. Highly active chemoimmunotherapy cisplatin IL-2 alfa interferon (IFN) in the treatment of metastatic malignant melanoma. Proc ASCO 1992; 11:353.

60. Legha S, Plager C, Ring S et al. A phase II study of biochemotherapy using

interleukin-2 (IL-2) plus interferon alfa-2A (IFN) in combination with cisplatin, vinblastine and DTIC in patients with metastatic melanoma. Proc ASCO 1992; 11:343

61. Richards J, Mehta N, Schroeder L, Dordal A. Sequential chemotherapy/immunotherapy for metastatic melanoma. Proc ASCO 1992; 11:346.

62. Tchekmedyian NS, Tait N, Van Echo D, Aisner J. High-dose chemotherapy without autologous bone marrow transplantation in melanoma. J Clin Oncol 1986; 4:1811-18.

63. Shea TC, Antman KH, Eder JP. Malignant melanoma: Treatment with high-dose combination alkylating agent chemotherapy and autologous bone marrow support. Arch Dermatol 1988; 124:878-84.

64. Thatcher N, Lind M, Morgenstern G et al. High-dose, double alkylating agent chemotherapy with DTIC, melphalan, or ifosfamide and marrow rescue for metastatic malignant melanoma. Cancer 1989; 63:1296-1302.

65. Wolff SN, Herzig RH, Fay JW et al. High-dose thiotepa with autologous bone marrow transplantation for metastatic malignant melanoma: results of phase I and II studies of the North American Bone Marrow Transplantation Group. J Clin Onc 1989; 7:245-9.

66. Lakhani S, Selby P, Bliss JM et al. Chemotherapy for malignant melanoma: combinations and high doses produce more responses without survival benefit. Br J Cancer 1990; 61:330-4.

67. Meisenberg B, Ross M, Jones R et al. Adjuvant high-dose combination alkylating agent chemotherapy (HDCAA) with autologous bone marrow support (ABMS) in multi-node positive melanoma. Proc ASCO 1992; 11:345.

CHAPTER 8

IMMUNOTHERAPY AND BIOLOGICAL THERAPY OF MALIGNANT MELANOMA

Evan M. Hersh, Charles W. Taylor
and Stanley P.L. Leong

Malignant melanoma has been of considerable interest as a potential target for immunotherapy and biological therapy for many decades. Initially, interest in melanoma as a target for immunotherapy derived from several important clinical observations. These included the observation of spontaneous regressions in malignant melanoma and the observation that lymphocytic infiltration of the primary tumor was associated with a better prognosis than when the primary tumor was not infiltrated with lymphocytes.[141] These both suggested a role for host defense factor in response to the development of melanoma.

Malignant melanoma was also one of the first malignancies in which both cellular and humoral anti-tumor immune responses were documented in man. Cellular immune responses included delayed type hypersensitivity (DTH) skin test reactions to the injection of melanoma extracts, cytotoxic activity of melanoma patient lymphocytes in killing melanoma cells in vitro, and lymphocyte proliferative responses to autologous melanoma cells or melanoma cell extracts.[77] Humoral immune responses were also observed and included the demonstration of cytotoxic antibodies to autologous melanoma in the serum of melanoma patients.[124] These observations, and their extensions described below provide the rationale and scientific basis for immunotherapy and biological therapy of malignant melanoma.

The development of monoclonal antibody technology has also had a profound impact on our understanding of the immunobiology of malignant melanoma. It has added to the data base supporting the hypothesis that immunotherapy of malignant melanoma would have clinical activity. Initially, several murine monoclonal antibodies to malignant melanoma cells were developed.[46] The majority of these reacted with melanoma associated antigens on the tumor cell surface, although some also reacted with internal melanoma associated antigens. These murine monoclonal antibodies identified melanoma associated antigens expressed predominantly, but not exclusively on melanoma cells. The majority of antigens identified with murine monoclonal antibodies had a low-level of representation on normal human tissues of various sites of origin. However they sometimes identified other tumors such as neutroblastoma.[16]

The murine monoclonal antibodies tended to identify glycoprotein, glycolipid, and ganglioside antigens. Subsequently, some of these monoclonal antibodies were utilized in studies of radioimmunolocalization, using antibodies coupled to Indium[111], Iodine[131] or Technetium[99] and have also been used for immunotherapy with antibodies coupled to chemotherapeutic agents, radioactive isotopes, cytokines, toxins or used unmodified. In the latter case, the antibodies mainly were those mediating antibody dependent cell-mediated cytotoxicity (ADCC) or complement-mediated lysis. These will be described in detail below.

Subsequent to the development of murine monoclonal antibodies, human monoclonal antibodies to malignant melanoma were also developed.[54] The latter proved that humans could make antibody to their own melanoma cells, adding strength to the concept that malignant melanoma induces an immune response in the tumor bearing subject. Such antibodies would be ideal candidates for the development of immunotherapy based on specificity and presumed lack of toxicity.

More recently, related to the development of lymphokine-activated killer cell (LAK cell) and tumor infiltrating lymphocyte (TIL) therapy of malignant melanoma, more extensive work on cytotoxic T-cell reactions to malignant melanoma have been carried out.[19] Important data include the observation that in ocular melanoma, the V-alpha gene region utilization of the T-cell receptor is highly restricted.[100] In addition, the cytotoxic T-cell lines have been utilized to identify specific melanoma associated antigens recognized by cytotoxic T-cells and at least one of these antigens has now been sequenced and its gene cloned.[148] Thus, not only are the cellular and humoral immune responses to malignant melanoma antigens being recognized but also the recognized antigens are also being characterized at the molecular level. These antigens will ultimately be used in therapeutic vaccines.

An important aspect of immune recognition in malignant melanoma relates to HLA-I antigen expression. In experimental murine systems, immune recognition of autologous tumor requires H-2 antigen presentation of tumor associated antigens.[113] In human malignant melanoma there appears to be a correlation between the presence of HLA antigen expression on tumor cells and a good prognosis; or the converse, the lack of expression HLA antigens and a poor prognosis.[126] In animal systems H-2 antigen transfection into tumor cells has been shown to increased their immunogenicity.[101] This in turn has led to the initiation of proposals for gene therapy experiments in human malignant melanoma involving transfection of HLA antigens into the malignant tumor.

In addition to lymphocyte and antibody-mediated host-defense mechanisms, there is also evidence that activated monocytes or macrophages may mediate antitumor host defense. In vitro, activated monocytes can kill autologous melanoma cells.[14] Consequently, monocyte activation is also a potential mechanism to be exploited for immunotherapy for malignant melanoma.

HISTORICAL PERSPECTIVE

From a historical prospective, the modern era of immunotherapy of malignant melanoma began in late 60s. Nonspecific immune activation was applied directly (topical or intralesional) to local melanoma nodules and induced regression therein. The nonspecific immune activators used at the time included *Bacillus Calmette Guerin* (BCG) and dinitrochlorobenzene (DNCB). Both of these agents induced nonspecific delayed type hypersensitivity and inflammatory responses within the tumor.[14] These responses included the infiltration of lymphocytes and monocytes which were felt to mediate tumor cell destruction, in part by a so called "bystander effect". The mechanism of this effect was not understood at the time. It was hypothesized that direct tumor cell killing by membrane interactions of effector with target cells and the release of cytotoxic molecules from the effector cells both played a role.

These early studies prompted a series of clinical experiments in which nonspecific immune activators such as BCG, *Corynebacterium parvum* (C. parvum), and other microbial adjuvants were given by several routes including intralesionally, regionally in the tumor lymph node drainage, and systematically for the therapy of melanoma. In addition to intact microbial organisms, microbial extracts and fractions were also used. Most of this work was based on extensive animal tumor modeling, particularly in the guinea pig tumor model.[157] In this model, tumor was inoculated into the flank and metastasized to regional lymph nodes. Intralesional BCG caused regression of both primary disease and disease in regional lymph nodes. It also conferred a strong immunity against rechallenge with the same tumor.

Concurrent with the investigation of nonspecific microbial adjuvants, a limited amount of clinical work was also begun with immunomodulators. Immunomodulators may be defined as drugs which augment or restore depressed immune responses, down-regulate hyperactive immune responses, and modulate or normalize perturbed or "out of balance" immune responses. In a variety of malignancies, there was a progressive decline in immunocompetence with progressive disease.[39] Furthermore, this was accentuated by immunosuppressive effects of surgery, radiation, and chemotherapy. A strong correlation was noted between immunocompetence and prognosis. It was hypothesized that in advanced metastatic malignant melanoma, general immune deficiency or immunosuppression of this type could be reversed by immunomodulators, while in early malignant melanoma, there might be specific antimelanoma responses which were down-regulated and which could be restored by immunomodulation. Therefore studies with immunomodulatory drugs such as thymic hormones[109] and levamisole[115] were done.

Also during this period of time, the earliest studies with tumor cell vaccines, utilizing allogeneic tumor cell lines and autologous tumor cells to augment specific anti-tumor immunity were initiated.[153]

Subsequently, advances in this field, involving cytokine therapy and monoclonal antibodies have related to modern advances in technology, namely the development of gene cloning and the production of genetically engineered cytokines such as interferon-α (IFN-α)[58] and interleukin-2 (IL-2)[36] and the development of hybridoma methodology. These now constitute the main thrust of modern research in immunotherapy of melanoma.

TECHNICAL AND SCIENTIFIC ADVANCES

Three major scientific and technical advances have moved the immunotherapy and biological therapy of malignant melanoma into the modern era. The first of these was the development of genetic engineering and the production of human cytokines, such as IFN-a and IL-2 by recombinant DNA technology. This has led first to the development of IFN-a therapy for malignant melanoma and other tumors.[58] It has also led to the discovery of the IL-2 driven LAK cell phenomenon,[30] and subsequently the development of IL-2 plus LAK cell therapy,[121] IL-2 therapy

alone,[41] IL-2 plus TIL cell therapy,[123] and to the development of research protocols with interleukin-1 (IL-1),[104] interleukin-4 (IL-4),[92] and interleukin-6 (IL-6).[149] All may be useful in the treatment of malignant melanoma. The development of recombinant cytokines has also greatly accelerated research on cytotoxic T-cells to malignant melanoma and on the structures recognized by cytotoxic T-cells.[148]

The second advance was the development of hybridoma and monoclonal antibody technology.[84] Both murine and human monoclonal antibodies have been developed to melanoma associated antigens on human malignant melanoma cells. These have been used to define the melanoma associated antigens and are currently under investigation, preclinically and clinically, as diagnostic and therapeutic tools for the management of malignant melanoma.

The third major advance is the development of methods to transfect mammalian cells with genes which are subsequently expressed by these cells.[57] This will form the basis of gene therapy in which genetically altered autologous or allogeneic cells will be administered as vaccines.

APPROACH TO IMMUNOTHERAPY AND BIOLOGICAL THERAPY

One of the principles espoused for cancer immunotherapy and biological therapy is that it should be most active in states of minimal residual disease, and that it should be utilized as adjuvant therapy after maximum tumor burden reduction has been achieved by surgery, radiation, or chemotherapy.[103] It is of interest in regard to this often espoused hypothesis that in fact, the efficacy of immunotherapy and biological therapy in malignant melanoma as well as in other malignant diseases has been mainly demonstrated in patients with measurable, locally recurrent or metastatic disease. Thus, efficacy of BCG, IFN-α, IFN-γ, IL-2, LAK cells, TIL cells, IL-1, and tumor cell vaccines have all been demonstrated in patients with metastatic disease.

While a limited number of reports, including some prospectively randomized control trials, suggest that immunotherapy and biological therapy may be active in the adjuvant setting, there is no fully confirmed observation in this regard. Adjuvant therapy with biological response modifiers remains entirely experimental in melanoma at this time. However, in experimental systems, immunotherapy and biological therapy are more active in limited disease, and therefore this area of research should continue to receive high priority among clinical investigators. It is imperative however that the studies be prospective randomly.

For example, the Southwest Oncology Group recently completed a randomized study of adjuvant IFN-γ in stage I and II malignant melanoma.[31] There was a basis of preclinical and clinical data on which to predict that IFN-γ would be effective adjuvant therapy. Unfortunately, no significant prolongation of disease-free interval or survival was noted. The Southwest Oncology Group is currently conducting randomized studies of the adjuvant use of IFN-α in two-dosage schedules and of allogeneic melanoma cell vaccine (Melacine), both directed at preventing recurrence in patients with stage

I or II disease rendered NED by surgery. Limited studies using interferon,[18] tumor cell vaccines,[110] or levamisole[115,134] reporting positive results need further confirmation in larger numbers of patients.

Several different classifications of the immunotherapy and biological therapy of cancer have been developed over the years. The classification given below is a practical one which we have found useful and which is specifically relevant to the current status of immunotherapy and biological therapy of malignant melanoma.

ACTIVE NONSPECIFIC IMMUNOTHERAPY

This modality of treatment was the first to be used in the management of melanoma. It refers to the administration of agents which activated or stimulated general host response mainly of an inflammatory type. We now know that such nonspecific maneuvers induce cytokines and activate specific host defense mechanisms. Most active, nonspecific immunotherapeutic agents are microbial organisms, their extracts or fractions.

Historically, the first major approach to the immunotherapy of malignant melanoma has been active nonspecific immunotherapy. It mainly utilized microbial adjuvants such as BCG and *C. parvum*, but also nonspecific inflammatory stimuli such as DNCB. A wide variety of intact microbial organisms, both intact viable and killed or extracted were also utilized.[38] None have stood the test of time, certainly not in melanoma, and none have developed into accepted modalities of treatment.

Clinical studies were based on earlier work in animal models in which it was shown that BCG immunotherapy could increase the resistance to subsequently inoculated malignant cells.[4] The use of active nonspecific immunotherapeutic agents was initially applied locally by topical (DNCB), or intralesional (BCG) therapy.[112] At the time these studies were started (in the late 1960s and early 1970s), specific mechanisms were not understood, however it was assumed that lymphocytes and monocytes or macrophages, participating in a delayed type hypersensitivity reaction to the applied agent, would kill tumor cells by direct contact or through the release of toxic substances. At that time, such cytotoxic cytokines were not yet identified, but were subsequently shown to include IFN-α, IFN-γ, TNF, and lymphotoxin.

In the initial report local immunotherapy resulted in regression of the treated nodule in approximately two-thirds of the cases and regression of untreated nodules in the same patients, after local immunotherapy, was noted in about 20% of the cases.[112] Of interest, only patients who where immunocompetent, by virtue of having intact delayed type hypersensitivity responses, remitted. Those patients who were immunoincompetent failed to remit.

Over 20 studies using BCG, the methanol extraction residue of BCG (MER), purified protein derivative of tubercle bacilli (PPD), and DNCB have been reported, with the response rates of the locally inoculated tumor varying from approximately 20% to as high as 80% or more.[90] Generally, toxicity was limited to a local reaction which could be severe including ulceration, and moderate systemic symptoms such as fever, chills, and flu-like symptoms. There continues to be a very limited role in clinical practice for the intralesional injection of BCG into symptomatic melanoma nodules which cannot be managed by conventional modalities. This approach can control local disease effectively but does not alter ultimate outcome. It is not FDA approved for this indication but only for the topical therapy of superficial recurrent bladder cancer.

These initial studies of local intratumoral BCG inoculation inspired attempts to use BCG immunotherapy by systemic administration. BCG was administered by scarification, usually applied sequentially on a weekly or twice monthly schedule by rotation to the upper and lower extremities.[32] BCG was used as adjuvant therapy after the surgical extirpation of stage I and II disease,[32] or was combined with chemotherapy for patients with advanced metastatic disease.[33]

Initial reports were that the disease-free interval after surgery and the survival were prolonged in BCG recipients.[32] The duration of response to chemotherapy for metastatic disease was reported to be prolonged in the BCG recipients compared to controls.[33] However, the majority of these early studies were done using historical controls. In prospectively randomized trials, efficacy of BCG in these types of studies was generally marginal and long-term survival was not effected.[150] Similar observations were made using active nonspecific immunotherapy with MER[43] and *C. parvum*.[145]

Today, physicians still use intralesional BCG to a very limited extent to treat local disease (although this is not FDA approved). The use of BCG and other active nonspecific active immunotherapeutic agents for systemic therapy to prevent relapse or treat metastatic disease has not been continued. It is to be emphasized that even for local treatment by intralesional injection, there is no evidence that overall survival of patients with metastatic disease is prolonged.

ACTIVE SPECIFIC IMMUNOTHERAPY (VACCINES)

Active specific immunotherapy involves vaccines to induce or augment an in vivo antimelanoma response in the melanoma bearing patient. Immunogens include autologous tumor cells, allogenic tumor cells, vaccines derived from extraction of melanoma cell surface structures such as glycoprotein or ganglioside antigens and anti-idiotype immunoglobulins. Anti-idiotype antibody presents the internal image of an antimelanoma monoclonal antibody which then mimics the immunogenic epitope of the tumor antigen. The use of adjuvants to augment the specific immune responses to the melanoma cell surface structures is an important component of this approach.

The use of melanoma vaccines is based on multiple observations of tumor-associated or tumor-specifics cell mediated immunity to malignant melanoma.[52] Cytotoxic reactions of lymphocytes against melanoma cells using lymphocytes derived from melanoma patients and autologous or allogeneic target melanoma cells were reported as long ago as 15 years. As the nature of the cytotoxic T-lymphocyte in anti-tumor host defense became characterized, numerous reports of cytotoxic T-lymphocytes killing autologous tumor cells have appeared.[2] Most recently, the ability to grow tumor infiltrating lymphocytes has resulted in populations of

clone cytotoxic T-cells with specificity for autologous tumor.[53,68] Indeed the antigens recognized by cytolytic T-lymphocytes on human malignant melanoma have been identified and purified and most recently genes encoding at least one of these antigens have been isolated.[148] In past years and continuing on until the present, multiple reports that patients with melanoma had cytotoxic antibodies in their serum to their own melanoma cells have also appeared.[151] It was show that immunization with tumor cells or tumor antigens can induce increased levels of these cytotoxic antibodies in patients with melanoma.[71] Thus there is a strong rational basis for the use of melanoma vaccines to prevent the recurrence of melanoma after primary surgery or to treat metastatic disease.

A number of preliminary reports in small numbers of patients have indeed demonstrated the potential degree of efficacy of this approach. Various types of melanoma vaccines have been used. These have included intact autologous melanoma cells, allogeneic melanoma cells, vaccinia lysates of allogeneic melanoma cells, Newcastle disease virus lysates of allogeneic melanoma cells, melanoma cell extracts, supernatants of cultured melanoma cells, purified melanoma associated antigens, and anti-idiotype monoclonal antibodies expressing the internal image of murine antimelanoma antibodies. A number of these studies have been Phase I and have shown the induction of cytotoxic T-cells and cytolytic antibodies.[71] A number, usually involving a small number of patients, have been Phase II and have documented responses. Clinical responses have been seen to autologous melanoma cells,[6] allogeneic melanoma cell extracts,[70] allogeneic melanoma cell viral oncolysates[98] and have mainly been partial remissions. The response rates in small numbers of patients have been between 10 and 20%. An important aspect of work with melanoma vaccines is the use of adjuvants or immunomodulators. Extensive studies based on appropriate animal model work had been done with low dose cyclophosphamide. Low dose cyclophosphamide abrogates suppressor cell activity and augments both cellular and humoral immune responses to vaccines.[9] In one study in which the immunogen was the GM-2 ganglioside, responses were significantly more vigorous when immunization was proceeded with cyclophosphamide then when it was not.[71] Other adjuvants have included BCG[8] and the unique modified endotoxin DETOX.[85]

Clearly, more extensive studies including randomized controlled trials need to be done with melanoma vaccines. The biology of the response to the vaccine should be studied in order to determine the characteristics of the responders and non-responders, both in terms of the patient and in terms of the vaccine. Increased antigen expression, increased immunogenecity, polyvalent vaccines, immunomodulation and appropriate adjuvants should all be explored in depth. Purified tumor associated or tumor specific antigens offer perhaps the best prospect. These include the HMW-HAA anti-idiotype molecule,[87] purified GM-2 ganglioside,[49] purified GM-3, GD-2 and GD-3 ganglioside[71] and the newly cloned and expressed tumor specific antigen recognized by cytotoxic T-lymphocytes (MZ2-E).[148] It will also be important to explore the relationship of HLA antigen expression to the immunogenecity of vaccines because presumably unique antigens will be expressed selectively by specific HLA molecules.

REGIONAL IMMUNOTHERAPY

In malignant melanoma regional therapies are important modalities. Regional surgery, radiation and regional chemotherapy such as perfusion are important ways of controlling disease. Regional immunotherapy with either intralymphatic or intralesional administration of BCG, the interferons, or TNF are approaches of some effect on local regional metastases but not on systemic disease or on ultimate outcome.

MONOCLONAL ANTIBODIES

Both murine and human antimelanoma monoclonal antibodies are used in experimental immunotherapy of melanoma. These antibodies, directed at tumor cell surface antigens are used neat and also as conjugates coupled to drugs, isotopes, cytokines or toxins which target cytotoxic substances to tumor cells.

Since the discovery of the monoclonal antibody technology in 1975 murine monoclonal antibodies have been produced which recognize a wide variety of tumor associated antigens on human and animal malignant tumors. In the case of malignant melanoma these antigens include peptideoglycans such as 9.2.27[156] transferrin receptor related antigens such as 96.5,[12] glycoproteins,[47,51] high molecular weight melanoma associated antigens,[142] sialoglycoproteins, and gangliosides.[71,49]

Each of these antigens is a cell-surface antigen which would be accessible to circulating monoclonal antibodies in vivo. An interesting feature of these antibodies is that the antigens they recognize do not have 100% representation on all tumor cells in a tumor nodule. Therefore, it has been proposed and documented that a higher proportion of tumor cells would be recognized by cocktails of monoclonals.[62] In addition, it was hypothesized and subsequently proven that expression of some of these antigens can be upregulated by exposure to cytokines such as IFN–α and IFNγ.[76] This suggested a potential role for combination monoclonal antibody therapy.

Theoretically, monoclonal antibodies can be utilized neat or coupled to isotopes, cytotoxic drugs, cytokines, or toxins. Those coupled to isotopes can be used for external scanning and those coupled to all of these ligands can be used for therapy. Extensive studies have been done in malignant melanoma for radioimmunolocalization of metastatic disease using monoclonal antibodies coupled to radioactive isotopes including indium[111], iodine[131] and technetium.[99] These studies have shown a reasonable degree of localization in melanoma nodules.[97] Biopsies have shown persistence of antibody for some days within the tumor and a favorable tumor to normal tissue ratio.[63] However, there are major problems with radioimmunolocalization and this approach has yet to be accepted as a useful diagnostic tool. Some of the problems associated with this technique include the fact that only tumors greater than about 1-2 cm will image.[99] Small tumors do not image, brain tumors do not image and it

is frequently impossible to see hepatic metastasis because of the extremely high nonspecific uptake of the radio-labeled antibody in the liver.[99] Thus, at the present time this technique offers no advantage over conventional tumor imaging techniques. The nonspecific uptake in liver and reticuloendothelial system, as well as bone marrow, also suggests the potential for a high degree of toxicity when these monoclonal antibodies are coupled to cytotoxic drugs or radioactive isotopes.

In addition to using monoclonal antibodies as direct therapeutic agents or as carriers to target therapeutic agents to tumor cells, there is an additional approach to the use of monoclonal antibodies in the treatment of melanoma. Anti-idiotype antibodies reflecting the internal image of the antimelanoma monoclonal antibodies present a structure which mimics the tumor associated antigen.[87] Immunization with anti-idiotypes to the high molecular weight melanoma associated antigen (HMW MAA) have been carried out and regressions were seen in 3 out of 14 patients who developed antibody in one study.[87] Also in this study, those patients who developed antibody had a significantly longer survival than those who did not.

Three mechanisms have been hypothesized to explain the potential anti-tumor activity of monoclonal antibodies. They can mediate antibody dependent cell-mediated cytotoxicity (ADCC). They can facilitate, complement-mediated lysis of target cells and they can induce anti-idiotype antibody responses which in turn induce an antitumor antibody response in the patient. Anti-idiotype antibodies to murine monoclonals have been found in patients receiving monoclonal antibodies for diagnosis or therapy of malignant melanoma.

Relatively limited numbers of studies of monoclonal antibody therapy of melanoma have been carried out. One reviewer has pointed out that when the antibodies are used alone, those directed against glycolipids (namely gangliosides) seem to have more activity than those directed against the other antigens.[137] Monoclonal antibody 3F8 directed against the GD-2 ganglioside has resulted in 7 out of 17 patients with melanoma or neuroblastoma, showing partial remissions.[15] Monoclonal antibody R-24 initially showed 3 out 12 and later 4 out of 21 patients responding with partial remissions.[147] In one study, regression of cutaneous nodules were shown when anti-GD2 monoclonal antibody was injected directly intralesionally.[50]

In addition to murine monoclonal antibodies, human monoclonal antibodies are now being developed. They may play an important role in that they will be nonimmunogenic. One was shown to cause regression of human melanoma innoculated into the nude mouse.[156]

An approach to reducing the immunogenicity of murine monoclonal antibodies is to chimerize or humanize them. Phase I studies of such antibodies have been conducted and indeed they elicit less of a human anti-mouse antibody (HaMA) response.[127]

Major problems exist for the full development of monoclonal antibodies against malignant melanoma. These include the immunogenicity of mouse antibodies. The patients ultimately develop antibodies which neutralize the ability of the mouse antibody to bind to the tumor cell. This can also cause severe allergic reactions. The low affinity and nonspecificity of uptake of all anti-tumor monoclonal antibodies that have been studied clinically presents a major problem in terms of toxicity to normal tissues. For example, the Ricin A chain immunotoxin studies have shown a severe degree of toxicity in human recipients during the Phase I protocol.[135] The lack of melanoma associated antigen expression on all melanoma cells within a metastatic nodule and the heterogeneous expression of melanoma associated antigens from nodule to nodule also provide major obstacles. The latter could be overcome if a high energy radioisotope was coupled to the monoclonal since that would kill adjacent cells as well as the monoclonal antibody binding cells. In other systems it has been shown that monoclonal antibodies binding to the surface of tumor cells can down-regulate expression of the target antigen.[13] This is a theoretical problem but has not yet been demonstrated in human melanoma.

With the development of genetic engineering techniques, it has become feasible that many of these obstacles can be overcome. Humanized or human monoclonal antibodies can overcome immunogenicity. Mutation of antibody genes in genetic engineering systems can increase affinity and specificity. Cocktails of monoclonal antibodies can recognize more tumor cells than single monoclonal antibodies and cytokines can up-regulate the expression of tumor associated antigens. The application of some of these approaches may allow monoclonal antibodies to become useful agents in the therapy of malignant melanoma.

The integrins play an important role in invasion and metastasis of melanoma cells. Elevated expression of certain integrins or their receptors may be associated with lower invasion.[111] In contrast the vitronectin receptor is positively associated with invasiveness of melanoma presumably through interaction with its substrate and the induction of the expression of metalloproteinases such as the matrix degrading proteinase, type 4 collagenase.[128] Since integrins and their receptors are expressed on the tumor cell surface, they should be readily accessible to ligands which bind them and therefore may serve as a target, for example, for monoclonal antibodies or other molecules which could play a role in the immunotherapy or biological therapy of melanoma. In one study, a synthetic peptide sequence (GRGDS) was co-injected with B-16 melanoma cells and found to markedly inhibit the formation of pulmonary metastasis when these cells were injected into C-57B6 mice.[45] This confirms the potential of this approach to biological therapy.

CYTOKINE THERAPY

Cytokines are defined as proteins produced by cells in response to stimuli which mediate the cells' effector functions at a distance. Cytokines may be directly or indirectly toxic to tumor cells.

Cytokines, produced by genetic engineering, are the most extensively investigated biological therapeutic agents for melanoma at this time. These include the interferons, IFN-α, interferon-β (IFN-β) and interferon-γ (IΦN–γ), IL-2 alone or combined with IL-2-induced in vitro expanded LAK or TIL cells, other interleukins including IL-1, IL-4, and IL-6, and other cytokines including macrophage

colony stimulating factor (M-CSF) and tumor necrosis factor (TNF). Cytokines may act directly to kill or inhibit tumor cells or indirectly via host-defense activation.

Interferons

The interferons have potential for activity in malignant melanoma based on their direct cytostatic and cytotoxic activity to tumor cells, their capacity to activate host defense mechanisms such as NK cell and macrophage mediated cytotoxicity and their ability to alter tumor cells by upregulating HLA and tumor antigen expression.[3] Natural and recombinant interferons have been used in the treatment of malignant melanoma since the early 1980s. In spite of numerous studies of interferons alone and in combination with chemotherapy, their role in the management of melanoma is still not entirely clear. Limited studies with IFN-γ[34] and IFN-β[1] suggests that they have minimal activity in patients with metastatic disease. Reported response rates have ranged to zero to approximately 10%.

There has been one carefully designed study of IFN-γ as adjuvant treatment after surgery for patients with stage I and II disease.[81] In this study, not only was there no prolongation of the disease-free interval or survival but in fact there was a trend (statistically non-significant) towards a shorter disease-free interval and survival in the treated patients compared to the controls.

Over the last 12 years, studies of the treatment of metastatic malignant melanoma with IFN-α have been conducted with the cytokine used as a single agent or combined with single agent chemotherapy cisplatin (cDDP) or imidazole carboxamide (DTIC) or with combination chemotherapy. There has not been a rational and consistent design of these studies in terms of dose or schedule of IFN−α or in terms of timing of the IFN−α and the chemotherapy in the combined modality studies. IFN−α doses have ranged from as little as 1 MU 3 times per week up to 15 MU/m² of body surface area daily. The few comparative studies done often compare chemotherapy to chemotherapy plus IFN−α rather than IFN−α alone vs. IFN−α plus chemotherapy. This makes it hard to fully define the role of ιντερφερον alone. In addition, the numbers of patients in these studies are too small for firm conclusions to be drawn even when apparent differences are noted. For example, one group[26] reported a 53% response rate in patients receiving DTIC plus high-dose IFN−α vs. 20% in patients receiving DTIC alone. However, while significantly different, the confidence intervals of these two regimens overlapped. Overall response rates to IFN−α alone or with chemotherapy in the various reported studies have ranged from 0% up to approximately 50% and response durations from 4 to 6 months up to 12 to 14 months.[17,26,66,79,94] A reasonable summation of this work is that IFN−α alone induces a response rate of approximately 10–20% and about one-quarter of the responses are complete remissions. Responses have been most common in skin, lymph node and pulmonary metastases. Other visceral sites of disease such as hepatic metastases are much less responsive. Response durations are approximately six months or less.

As noted elsewhere in this review, the most promising use of IFN−α therapy appears to relate to its addition to combination chemotherapy. This has yielded response rates in the range of 60% and response durations in the range of 12 months.[29,67] However, comparative trials involving large numbers of patients have not been done and the conclusion that combined chemotherapy with high dose IFN−α or high dose IFN−α plus IL-2 is superior to chemotherapy alone or, in fact, to high-dose IFN−α alone cannot be made at this time.

Questions to be asked include the following. What is the optimal dose of IFN−α for response induction; what is the optimal schedule of IFN−α treatment (e.g. daily vs. 3 x per week); what is the optimal chemotherapy to be combined with IFN−α; should the IFN−α therapy precede, follow or be concurrent with the chemotherapy? As the incidence of melanoma increases dramatically, and as we are seeing more and more patients with this disease, the answers to these questions become extremely important. It is really mandatory at this point that we try to define the optimal state-of-the-art treatment for metastatic malignant melanoma. This can only be done using large numbers of patients in prospectively randomized trials; presumably conducted by one or more of the national cooperative groups.

The toxicity of IFN−α in malignant melanoma is similar to the toxicity of this drug as seen in other diseases.[114] The majority of patients will have mild fever and chills, flu-like symptoms, anorexia, fatigue, psychomotor retardation and weight loss. Most of the side effects can be readily distinguished from those of chemotherapy. However,

INF-α is myelosuppressive. Doses of 3 million units per day or more often result in mild to moderate myelosuppression with white counts in the range of 2500 to 3000 and platelet counts in the range of 75,000 to 100,000. Obviously in combination with chemotherapy this degree of myelosuppression may pose a problem.

Finally, it is to be noted that IFN–α, while useful in the management of melanoma and FDA approved for other indications, is not FDA approved specifically by the FDA for melanoma therapy.

Interleukin-2

The discovery that IL-2 induced the activation and proliferation of cytotoxic promiscuous killer lymphocytes, hereafter referred to as lymphokine activated killer cells or LAK cells, has initiated an entirely new era in the field of immunotherapy.[30] Initially LAK cells were shown to have the capacity to kill autologous and allogenic tumor cells but not normal cells. This killing was referred to as "promiscuous" since it was not HLA restricted. After the in vitro demonstration of LAK cell activity, the administration of LAK cells plus IL-2 to tumor bearing animals demonstrated that several different tumor types including nonimmunogenic tumors could be controlled by this therapy.[78] It was also observed that the regressing tumors were infiltrated with lymphocytes presumably the administered LAK cells.[5] Shortly thereafter Rosenberg and coworkers demonstrated that patients receiving IL-2-stimulated and in vitro-expanded LAK cells, plus high dose IL-2 (100,000 units per kg every 8 hours) experienced a substantial proportion of remissions. Responses were seen in patients with malignant melanoma, renal cell carcinoma, colon cancer and lymphoma.[121] This initial observation resulted in extensive studies of IL-2 and adoptive cellular immunotherapy over the last seven years.

IL-2 therapy can be classified into several categories in relationship to malignant melanoma:

1. High dose IL-2 plus autologous LAK cells.
2. High dose IL-2 alone.
3. Intermediate to low dose IL-2.
4. High dose IL-2 plus autologous tumor infiltrating lymphocytes.
5. Single agent or combination chemotherapy plus IL-2.

High dose IL-2 with or without LAK cells has elicited considerable controversy because of its confirmed activity and its extreme toxicity. Arguments in favor of high dose IL-2 therapy include the fact that it can induce some responses even in patients with advanced metastatic malignant disease and that in renal cell carcinoma it induces a very small proportion, less than 10% of long term remissions.[108] Based on this, high dose IL-2 therapy was recently approved by the FDA for the treatment of metastatic renal cell carcinoma. While showing some activity in malignant melanoma, long term complete remissions have been observed very rarely and therefore any use of IL-2 in malignant melanoma remains developmental. In spite of these concerns and limitations, various editorial reviewers have referred to IL-2 therapy as "immunotherapy the end of the beginning"[24] or "interleukin-2, sunrise for immunotherapy."[48]

While the initial report on high dose IL-2 with LAK cells reported response rates in the range of 50%[121] for melanoma, subsequent reports were less encouraging. The IL-2 LAK cell working group reported an overall response rate in melanoma of approximately 15%[75] while an update from the National Cancer Institute Group reported a CR + PR rate of 23% for LAK cells plus IL-2 and 31% for IL-2 alone.[123] These results were reported in a total of 42 patients. In a subsequent update involving a total of 90 patients, there were 21% responses among patients treated with IL-2 plus LAK cells of which somewhat less than half were complete remissions and 24% responses (all partial) among patients treated with high dose IL-2 alone.[122] Other groups have reported about a 22% response rate; mainly partial remissions in patients treated with the standard high dose IL-2 regimen.[107] Because of its toxicity, patient selection for high dose IL-2 therapy is very strict, excluding patients with an impairment of performance status or organ function and patients with large tumor burdens. Therefore, we can assume that the proportion of all metastatic melanoma patients who can benefit is quite small, certainly under 20%.

In addition to bolus IL-2, 100,000 units per kg every 8 hours, several groups have explored continuous infusion of IL-2 with or without LAK cells. The intent was to determine whether toxicity could be ameliorated by a different schedule of administration. Of interest, response rates and toxicity were similar to that described for the bolus injection, approximately 20% partial remissions and severe toxicity.[154]

After the initial observations with IL-2 plus LAK cells, Rosenberg and coworkers began to investigate the use of tumor infiltrating lymphocytes, so called TIL cells. Large numbers of these were generated by making cell suspensions from tumors and expanding the infiltrated lymphocytes in vitro by culture with IL-2. The hypothesis was that melanomas are infiltrated with cytotoxic T-cells which have HLA restricted specific cytotoxicity towards the autologous tumor. This hypothesis was partially supported by in vitro observations[52] and therefore subsequently clinical trials were initiated with IL-2 plus TIL cells. In the first report, a 50% response rate in malignant melanoma was noted.[123] Subsequently, in larger number of patients the response rate has been in the range of 35%[122] and in studies with IL-2 plus TIL cells reported by others, the response rate has been closer to 20 to 25%.[61,21] One group concluded that a treatment plan for IL-2 plus TIL cells is technically difficult, costly and effective for only a minority of patients.[22] Furthermore, overall clinical results are not clearly superior to those obtained with other regimens involving IL-2 as the only immunotherapeutic modality.

The next category of IL-2 therapy which has been investigated extensively includes the use of IL-2 at low to moderate doses which can be administered safely to outpatients either alone or combined with single agent or combination chemotherapy. IL-2 regimens included daily intravenous bolus injection, low dose continuous infusion, thrice weekly bolus injection, with treatment usually in periods of a one week on, one week off mode.

The studies in this class of treatment are very difficult to evaluate. Numbers of patients in each study are small. There is no consistency in dose or schedule from study to study. Few studies are randomized comparative trials. Timing of IL-2 therapy relative to chemotherapy in combined modality studies is highly variable. However, overall interpretation of these data is that the response rate to relatively low dose IL-2 therapy alone is in the range of 10-15%.[143] When IL-2 is combined with chemotherapy, there may be a slight degree of additive anti-tumor activity but not a major increase in the complete or partial remission rates compared to chemotherapy alone.[28]

Thus, all regimens of IL-2 treatment including high dose alone, high dose with LAK or TIL cells, low dose alone, and low dose plus chemotherapy should continue to be considered investigational. However, since IL-2 has now been approved for use in renal cell carcinoma, physicians are free to use it in the management of malignant melanoma. It can be recommended for patients in good physical condition, with normal performance status and no significant major organ disease such as cardiovascular disease. The use of IL-2 therapy can be considered for patients with metastatic disease as back-up or second/third line therapy. An occasional patient will have a very gratifying complete or major partial remission of long duration.

The major limitations on the use of IL-2 relates to its toxicity.[132] It is clear that high dose IL-2 is more active than low dose IL-2 but the severe toxicity limits its use. Approximately 5% of patients have had a fatal outcome usually related to myocardial infarction or arrhythmia.[122] High dose IL-2 induces a capillary leak syndrome with major shifts of fluid out of the vascular compartment.[125] This results in hypotension and prerenal azotemia requiring fluid restriction and treatment with pressors in the intensive care unit. Specific organ toxicities that have been observed include the following:[132] cardiovascular toxicity including arrhythmias, ischemia, infarction and myocarditis; nephrotoxicity including ischemia and oliguria; pulmonary edema with respiratory distress severe enough to require intubation and mechanical ventilation; nausea, vomiting and diarrhea; hepatocellular toxicity and intrahepatic cholestasis with hyperbilirubinemia; hypothyroidism; various skin eruptions; neurological toxicity including confusion, disorientation, hallucinations, somnolence and coma, and hematological toxicity including anemia and thrombocytopenia. Interestingly, there appears to be an increased incidence of bacterial infections in up to 30% of cases including disseminated cutaneous staphylococcal infections and bacterial sepsis.[96] The mechanisms of these toxicities are not clearly understood, but are felt to be related mainly to the capillary leak syndrome with marked changes in intracellular and extracellular fluid and electrolyte distribution causing the organ dysfunction. It is also hypothesized that this is the result of the release of other cytokines induced by IL-2 including TNF and lymphotoxin, and perhaps IL-1.[83] The release of nitric oxide as a mediator has been speculated to play a major role. This suggests that inhibitors of nitric oxide production such as Ng methyl L-arginine[102] could prevent IL-2 toxicity without altering its clinical anticancer activity. This is beginning to be explored in both in vitro and in vivo systems.

Other Cytokines

Several other interleukins and cytokines are of interest for the possible treatment of malignant melanoma. These include IL-1, IL-4, IL-6, M-CSF and TNF.

IL-1 may have direct anti-tumor activity and in addition can activate cytotoxic T-cells and LAK cells by increasing precursor cell IL-2 receptor expression.[23] IL-1 has direct cytotoxic activity against various tumor cell lines including A375 melanoma.[89] Its ability to increase expression of IL-2 receptors and to augment T lymphocyte mediated cytotoxicity and NK cell activity[25] could make it an active agent against melanoma. During a Phase I trial of IL-1, in patients with different malignancies, limited responses were seen in patients with malignant melanoma. Therefore, the number of patients being treated was extended. In the Phase I study, of 15 evaluable patients there was one CR and four PR's for an overall response rate of 33%.[136] It is to be pointed out, however, that IL-1 is one of the more toxic cytokines. Serious adverse side effects have included arrhythmias, pulmonary edema, hypotension, and bronchospasm, presumably related to the capillary leak syndrome. In spite of this, tolerable outpatient protocols for IL-1 have been developed and it is now in Phase II investigation.

IL-4 is a cytokine produced by activated T-cells which stimulates B-cell growth, T-cell proliferation, and augments human cytotoxic T lymphocyte proliferation after initial activation.[44] It also upregulates IL-2 receptors.[129] Therefore, it can also be expected to have activity in immunologically sensitive tumors. For this reason, it is undergoing Phase II investigation in malignant melanoma.

IL-6, a hematopoietic growth factor which stimulates hematopoietic progenerator proliferation and differentiation and induces the terminal differentiation and the release of platelets from megacaryocytes[72] also has immunological activity. It augments and increases the cytotoxic activity of T-cells and can also activate NK cell and ADCC mechanisms. It has been shown to be active in several murine tumor models and has direct proliferation inhibitory and differentiation inducing activity against human tumor cells in vitro[130] and in weakly immunogenic mouse tumor models.[95] It is currently undergoing Phase I evaluation in cancer patients.

TNF administered systemically does not induce remission in malignant melanoma.[40] However, there may be some role in its regional administration via the intraarterial route.[69]

RELATED APPROACHES

New approaches related to the above categories are receiving increasing attention. The purification and cloning of tumor antigens opens a new possibility for active vaccine development. Gene therapy in which tumor cells are transfected with selected genes and modified to express cytokines or antigens such as interleukins or HLA antigens is in both preclinical and clinical development. These modified cells are then used as vaccines. Finally, it is possible that the exploitation of cell adhesion molecules which play a critical role in the dissemination of malignant melanoma may also provide a target for effective biological therapy.

IMMUNOMODULATION

Studies of immunomodulation in melanoma have included the use of stimulators of T-cell proliferation or differentiation, such as levamisole and thymic hormones. Also drugs which modify suppressor cell activity such as cimetidine for suppressor T-cells and indomethacin for inhibition of suppressor macrophages belong in this category. Abrogation of suppressor cell activity theoretically augments specific antimelanoma responses. Low-dose cyclophosphamide has been used to down-regulate suppressor cell activity and to permit a more vigorous response to active specific immunization in melanoma.

Immunomodulation is based on the hypothesis that there is specific or general immunoincompetence in the melanoma patient and this incompetence permits the progression of immunogenetic melanoma. Immunocompetence and a good prognosis are directly related in cancer patients.[42] Therefore, restoration of the general immunocompetent by an immunomodulator would also restore the specific antimelanoma immunity which would in turn control the growth of the melanoma cells. All of the approaches to melanoma including the use of active nonspecific immunotherapeutic agents such as BCG, cytokines such as IFN−α, LAK cells and tumor vaccines can in as sense be considered immunomodulatory. However, here we use the term immunomodulation to refer to those drugs which can up-regulate suppressed immune responses or general immunocompetence. Several immuno-modulators have been used in malignant melanoma. Levamisole is an immunomodulatory imidazole compound which is of proven efficacy in combination with 5-fluorouracil in preventing recurrence of Dukes' Class C colon cancer after surgery.[88] Several studies of Levamisole as an immunomodulator to prevent recurrence and prolonged survival in malignant melanoma have been carried out. The data is conflicting and both negative[134] and positive[115] studies have been reported. Cimetidine has immunomodulatory properties in that it down-regulates H2 receptor bearing T-suppressor lymphocytes. Again reports of cimetidine's efficacy in malignant melanoma[138] have been counteracted by negative reports.[73] Indomethacin, an inhibitor of PGE_2 synthesis, theoretically can down-regulate the function of suppressor macrophages while Indomethacin has shown this activity in vitro,[133] no evidence exists for its in vivo activity in malignant melanoma. Low dose cyclophosphamide can down-regulate the action of suppressor T-cells during the immune response.[9] While there is some evidence that cyclophosphamide can augment the response to melanoma vaccines,[71] the appropriate trials to demonstrate unequivocally that cyclophosphamide can be active as an adjunct to melanoma immunotherapy have not been done. There are reports of the use of cyclophosphamide in combination with melanoma vaccines or in combination with cytokine therapy. Response rates in these studies are more or less similar to those done in the absence of cyclophosphamide.[105] Therefore, until large scale controlled trials are carried out, the role of cyclophosphamide remains completely speculative.

COMBINATION THERAPY

Combination therapy is an approach of growing importance. Combinations of biological agents with each other and with chemotherapy are both being investigated actively at the present time. The concept is one of additive anti-tumor activity without additive toxicity. For some combinations, synergy between the agents can be demonstrated in vitro.

Once it was observed that immunotherapeutic or biological therapy agents had some degree of activity alone in malignant melanoma (IFN-α, IL-2, LAK cells, TIL cells, monoclonal antibodies, or tumor cell vaccines), a logical extension was to use these therapeutic agents in combination with chemotherapy. A large number of studies have been reported recently combining 1) DTIC, 2) cDDP, 3) DTIC plus cDDP, 4) tamoxifen, carmustine (BCNU), DTIC plus cDDP, and other therapeutic regimens of chemotherapy with IFN-α, IL-2 alone, IL-2 plus LAK or TIL cells, IFN-α plus IL-2, etc. These studies will be detailed below.

Several hypotheses drive this work. These include the concept that chemotherapy and biological therapy would have non-overlapping toxicities. Therefore they could be combined at full-dose with additive therapeutic activity and without additive toxicity. A few preclinical studies indicate that chemotherapeutic and biological therapy agents act synergistically. For example, chemotherapy could make tumor cells more sensitive to the cytotoxic actions of effector cells or molecules.

However, with some exceptions, the clinical data generated thus far indicate a less than additive effect when chemotherapy and biological therapy are combined. In general, response rates response durations and survivals have not been increased compared to that induced by chemotherapy alone. This does not diminish the fact that IFN-α, IL-2, LAK and TIL cells, tumor cell vaccines and monoclonal antibodies all have measurable response rates in melanoma and that the small fraction of patients induced into complete remission with these agents generally have a prolonged survival compared to that which would be expected, or compared to that in patients not achieving complete remission.

Another factor that complicates the evaluation of these combined chemotherapy plus biological therapy regimens is that few of them have been randomized controlled studies utilizing large enough numbers of patients on which firm conclusions can be drawn.

Combined modality therapy for malignant melanoma includes the combination of chemotherapy with biological therapy, the combination of more than one modality of biological therapy, the use of chemomodulation preceding biological therapy and the combination of chemotherapy with chemomodulation. Many of the modalities of biological therapy including the interferons, interleukins, effector cells, tumor vaccines, monoclonal antibodies and immunomodulators have been used in combination with each other and with chemotherapy. The cytokines which have been combined with chemotherapy as single agents include IFN-α, β and γ, IL-2 and TNF.

Chemotherapy has also been combined both with IL-2 plus LAK cells, IL-2 plus TIL cells and IL-2 plus IFN-α. Rates of remission for the chemotherapy regimens used in these combinations previously reported (without the cytokines) have ranged from 15% to 50%. The response rates to the cytokines without chemotherapy have ranged in the reported series from 10% to 40%.

The numbers of studies combining chemotherapy with cytokines have increased substantially since recombinant cytokines became available in 1985. Thus, there were three studies in 1985 – 1986, five in 1987– 1988, and between ten and twelve per year were reported in 1989, 1990, 1991 and 1992. Several studies combining DTIC or other single agents with IFN-α have been reported.[11,26,37,55,56,59,80,82,93,146] The response rates have ranged from 0% to 53% in different studies. The overall response rate of 243 patients is 32%. Two randomized comparative studies have been done involving the total of 117 patients.[82,146] The response rate to DTIC alone was 25% and to DTIC plus IFN-a was 39%. Thus, there may be additive effect when interferon is added to DTIC. The dose of interferon may also influence the response. The CR plus PR rate for patients receiving interferon at 60 million units (MU) per week or lower was 0 to 22% in the reported studies compared to 30% to 53% in patients receiving on the average approximately 90 MU per week. In conclusion, IFN-a may add to DTIC therapy but this is certainly not a firm conclusion at this time and the advantage of using the combination appears to be modest.

Several studies report the combination of cDDP with IFN-α. A total of 53 patients had an overall response rate of 25%.[74,119] Four studies report a combination of DTIC and IL-2; patients had an overall response rate of about 25%.[20,27,131,139] Thus, single agent chemotherapy plus single agent cytokine therapy appears to offer little advantage to either alone.

Somewhat more encouraging results are seen when biological therapy is added to combination chemotherapy. In five studies, the response rates reported a range from 37% to 83% and there were 50% responses among 102 patients.[10,31,35,67,116] DTIC or cDDP plus IFN–α or IL-2 led to response rates in six studies ranging from 23% to 35% whereas two to four chemotherapy drugs combined with IFN–α and/or IL-2 in five studies gave an overall response rate of 50%. With chemotherapy alone, complete remission rates are low and the proportion of responding patients (CR plus PR) entering complete remission is usually around 10% to 20%. In the studies of combination chemotherapy plus cytokine therapy, this is somewhat higher and has ranged from 26% to 63% in the reviewed studies.

Another aspect of the combination of chemotherapy with biological therapy is the use of cyclophosphamide as an immunomodulator. The scientific basis for this approach is that cyclophosphamide treatment prevents high zone tolerance to sheep red blood cells in mice, reverses tumor-induced immunosuppression and has been shown to augment various immune responses in cancer patients including primary and recalled delayed hypersensitivity to microbial antigens, primary antibody response, lymphocyte proliferation and delayed hypersensitivity to tumor antigen.[7] Therefore, it is concluded that cyclophosphamide can act to augment or facilitate various types of immunotherapy particularly that involving a specific immune response. The presumed mechanism is down-regulation of suppressor cell activity.

A number of studies have been reported in which low immunomodulatory doses of cyclophosphamide have been added to IFN–α,[152] IL-2 therapy[86] or treatment with a monoclonal antibody Ricin A chain immunoconjugate.[106] In addition, cyclophosphamide immunomodulation has also been used with autologous and allogeneic tumor cell vaccines.[71] Response rates have ranged from 6% to 25% in these various studies. These are very similar response rates to those induced by the immunotherapeutic agent alone. At this point we would conclude that there is little data to establish the role of cyclophosphamide immunomodulation as either additive or synergistic with biological therapy for melanoma.

The most effective chemotherapy for malignant melanoma is the combination of tamoxifen (which presumably is acting as a chemomodifier), with BCNU, DTIC and cDDP. The response rate to this regimen is approximately 50% to 60%. Several have reported that this regimen followed by relatively high dose IL-2 and IFN–α given together has resulted in a response rate close to 60%.[67,118] Patients with very advanced disease and difficult sites such as hepatic metastases respond to this regimen. Patients entering complete remission on this regimen appear to have prolonged remission duration. Whether it is truly superior to the combination chemotherapy alone is not known and will have to be determined in prospectively randomized controlled studies. Such an effort would be worthwhile to clearly document the efficacy of this promising regimen.

There are several major questions to be answered in regard to the sequencing of combined chemotherapy and biological therapy. These questions could be approached through appropriate in vitro and animal model studies which would look at the influence of one therapy on the response to the subsequent therapy. Such studies might also detect whether sequential (chemotherapy followed by immunotherapy or immunotherapy followed by chemotherapy) or simultaneous administration had additive, synergistic or diminished effectiveness compared to either treatment alone. Unfortunately this has not been approached in either experimental systems or consistently in human studies. One group did report the apparent non-cross resistance of chemotherapy and immunotherapy (IFN–α + IL-2) in studies in which BCDT combination chemotherapy was administered to patients progressing after IL-2 treatment.[119] Fifty-five% of such patients responded which is equivalent to the response rate to BCDT reported in the literature. This simply suggests that chemotherapy and cytokine therapy are not cross resistant.

BONE MARROW TRANSPLANTATION

Another approach which can be considered biological therapy (as a form of adoptive cellular therapy) is bone marrow transplantation. High-dose chemotherapy followed by bone marrow transplantation (usually autologous) with or without immunorestorative therapy maneuvers is of some interests in melanoma at the present time.

High dose chemotherapy with autologous bone marrow rescue has been studied fairly extensively in patients with disseminated malignant melanoma.[60,64,140,144,155] The hypothesis being tested was that the complete remission and total remission rates would be increased thus prolonging survival. Various regimens of high dose combination chemotherapy have been administered, followed by autologous bone marrow transplantation. While the toxicity was high, bone marrow transplantation was effective in maintaining good survival in these patients. Response rates in excess of 80% with complete responses in the range of 30% have been observed in these studies. Unfortunately, the majority of studies show no major prolongation of overall survival, although a small subset of patients (perhaps in the 5–10%) have a survival >1 year.[60] At the present time, it can be concluded that high dose combination chemotherapy followed by autologous bone marrow transplantation is still experimental and may be useful but only in a small proportion of patients with relatively limited disseminated or metastatic disease.

CONCLUSIONS

The immunotherapy and biological therapy of malignant melanoma is now founded on an excellent scientific basis and shows promising preliminary results. The scientific basis includes the demonstration of melanoma associated antigens and tumor specific antigens in melanoma and their characterization, purification and cloning. It further includes the demonstration of both cellular and humoral tumor specific immune responses in melanoma. The development of human monoclonal antibodies to malignant melanoma is an important aspect of this proof.

The initial approaches to immunotherapy of malignant melanoma involved crude and uncharacterized reagents such as BCG and other microbial adjuvants. However, in recent years, we have seen the development of therapy for malignant melanoma involving recombinant DNA produced cytokines such as INFa and IL-2, LAK cells, partially cloned cytotoxic effector T-cells (TIL cells) and monoclonal antibodies directed against specific cell surfaced target molecules. In addition, early work with crude melanoma vaccines involving mixtures of allogenic tumor cells or tumor cell lysates is being replaced with vaccines consisting of purified or even cloned tumor-associated and tumor specific antigens. As the nature of the immune response to melanoma becomes further characterized, it is likely that even more specific immune manipulations will be approached clinically.

The fact that complete and partial remissions are induced in some patients with metastatic malignant melanoma by INFα, IL-2, LAK cells, TIL cells, tumor vaccines, etc. clearly indicates that there is already a role in clinical practice for the use of immunotherapy. The fact that the overall response rates to these maneuvers are in the range of 20% indicates that significant amount of additional and basic clinical research needs to be done with these approaches before they can be considered major additions to our armamentarium.

The combination of chemotherapy with biological therapy has also provided promising leads and chemotherapy plus cytokines or high dose chemotherapy plus bone marrow transplantation have resulted in response rates of 60% to 80% as opposed to the usual response rates of 20% to 40% with chemotherapy alone.

A major area waiting for the development is the use of immunotherapy and biological therapy as adjuvant treatment for the prevention of recurrence after surgical removal of stage I or stage II disease. While receiving considerable attention this area is yet to have a definitive lead showing enough promise for repeated multicenter studies.

One of the major problems in therapeutic research in malignant melanoma is the lack of a truly systematic approach and order in the design and conduct of clinical trials. What is meant by this, is that most studies are either not well controlled for comparing experimental to conventional therapy, involve too few patients meaningful conclusions can be drawn statistically, and are so highly variable in design from study to study in terms of dose, schedule, route and duration of therapy, that it is almost impossible to draw firm conclusions about the efficacy of a proposed approach. Therefore, we continue to suboptimally utilize clinical resources and significantly delay a progress in the management of this disease.

Given the fact that the incidence of melanoma is increasing throughout the world, it seems that with the scientific and early clinical advances outlined above, the organization and administration of logical approaches to therapeutic research in this disease should receive an extremely high priority.

REFERENCES

1. Abdi EA, Tan YH, McPherson TA. Natural human interferon-beta in metastatic malignant melanoma. A phase II study. Acta-Oncol 1988; 27:815-17.
2. Aebersold P, Hyatt C, Johnson S et al. Lysis of autologous melanoma cells by tumor-infiltrating lymphocytes: Association with clinical response. J Natl Cancer Inst 1991; 83:932-7.
3. Baron S, Tyring SK, Fleischmann Jr WR et al. The interferons. JAMA 1991; 266:1375-83.
4. Bartlett GL, Kreider JW. Animal models for evaluating therapeutic potential of immune stimulants. In: Hersh EM, Chirigos MA, Mastrangelo MJ, eds. Augmenting Agents in Cancer Treatment. New York: Raven Press, 1981:1-13.
5. Basse PH, Nannmark U, Johansson BR et al. Establishment of cell-to-cell contact by adoptively transferred adherent lymphokine-activated killer cells. J Natl Cancer Inst 1991; 83:944-50.
6. Berd D, Maguire Jr HC, Mastrangelo MJ. Induction of cell-mediated immunity to autologous melanoma cells and regression of metastases after treatment with a melanoma cell vaccine preceded by cyclophosphamide. Cancer Res 1986; 46:2572-7.
7. Berd D, Maguire Jr HC, Mastrangelo MJ. Potentiation of human cell-mediated and humoral immunity by low-dose cyclophosphamide. Cancer Res 1984; 44:5439-43.
8. Berd D, Maguire Jr HC, McCue P, Mastrangelo MJ. Treatment of metastatic melanoma with an autologous tumor-cell vaccine: Clinical and immunologic results in 64 patients. J Clin Oncol 8:1858-67 1990.
9. Berd D, Mastrangelo MJ. Active immunotherapy of human melanoma exploiting the immunopotentiating effects of cyclophosphamide. Cancer Investigation 1988; 6:337-349.

10. Blair S, Flaherty L, Valdivieso M, Redman B. Comparison of high dose interleukin-2 (HD IL-2) with combined chemotherapy/low dose IL-2 (CHEMO/IL-2) in metastatic malignant melanoma (MMM). Proc ASCO 10:294(1031) 1991. (Abstract)

11. Breier S, Pensel R, Roffe C et al. High dose DTIC with recombinant human interferon alpha 2 b (rhIFN2b) for the treatment of metastatic malignant melanoma (MMM). Proc ASCO 9:281(1090) 1990. (Abstract)

12. Brown JP, Woodbury RG, Hart CE et al. Quantitative analysis of melanoma-associated antigen p97 in normal and neoplastic tissue. Proc Natl Acad Sci 1981; 78:539-43.

13. Brown SL, Miller RA, Horning SJ et al. Treatment of B cell lymphoma with anti-idiotype antibodies alone and in combination with alpha interferon. Blood 1989; 3:651.

14. Chakraborty NG, Okino T, Stabach P et al. Adoptive transfer of activated human autologous macrophages results in regression of transplanted human melanoma cells in SCID mice. In Vivo 1991; 5:609-14.

15. Cheung NKV, Lazarus H, Miraldi FD et al. Ganglioside GD2 specific monoclonal antibody 3F8: A phase I study in patients with neuroblastoma and malignant melanoma. J Clin Oncol 1987; 5:1430-40.

16. Cheung NKV, Saarinen UM, Neely J et al. Monoclonal antibodies to a glycolipid antigen on human neuroblastoma cells Cancer Res 1985; 45:2642-9.

17. Cregan ET, Schaid DJ, Ahmann DL, Frytak S. Recombinant interferons in the management of advanced malignant melanoma. Updated review of five prospective clinical trials and long-term responders. Am J Clin Oncol 1988; 11:652-9.

18. Cupissol D, Guillot B, Stoebner A et al. Adjuvant therapy with interferon (IFN) alfa-2b on malignant melanoma patients after surgical excision of skin or lymph node recurrence: New evaluation. Proc ASCO 1991; 10:299(1048). (Abstract)

19. Darrow TL, Slingluff CL, Seigler HF. The role of HLA class I antigens in recognition of melanoma cells by tumor-specific cytotoxic T lymphocyts. J Immunol 1989; 142:3329-35.

20. Demchak PA, Mier JW, Robert NJ et al. Interleukin-2 and high-dose cisplatin in patients with metastatic melanoma: A pilot study. J Clinc Oncol 1991; 9:1821-30.

21. Dillman RO, Oldham RK, Barth NM et al. Recombinant interleukin-2 and adoptive immunotherapy alternated with dacarbazine therapy in melanoma: A national biotherapy study group trial. J Natl Cancer Inst 1990; 82:1345-9.

22. Dillman RO, Oldham RK, Barth NM et al. Continuous interleukin-2 and tumor-infiltrating lymphocytes as treatment of advanced melanoma. A national biotherapy study group trial. Cancer 1991; 68:1-8.

23. Dinarello CA. Biology of interleukin 1. FASEB J 1988; 2:108-15.

24. Durant JR. Immunotherapy of cancer: The end of the beginning? N Engl J Med 1987; 316:939.

25. Durum SK, Schmidt JA, Oppenheim JJ. Interleukin 1: An immunological perspective. Ann Rev Immunol 1985; 3:263.

26. Falkson CI, Falkson G, Falkson HC. Improved results with the addition of interferon alfa-2b to dacarbazine in the the treatment of patients with metastatic malignant melanoma. J Clin Oncol 1991; 9:1403-8.

27. Flaherty LE, Liu PY, Fletcher WS et al. Dacarbazine and outpatient interleukin-2 in treatment of metastatic malignant melanoma: Phase II Southwest Oncology Group trial. J Natl Cancer Inst 1992; 84:893-4.

28. Flaherty LE, Redman BG, Chabot GG et al. A phase I-II study of dacarbazine in combination with outpatient interleukin-2 in metastatic malignant melanoma. Cancer 1990; 65:2471-7.

29. Garbe C, Kreuser ED, Zouboulis CC et al. Combined treatment of metastatic melanoma with interferons and cytotoxic drugs. Semin Oncol 1992; 19:63-9.

30. Grimm EA, Mazumder A, Zhang HZ, Rosenberg SA. Lymphokine-activated killer cell phenomenon: Lysis of natural killer-resistant fresh solid tumor cells by interleukin 2-activated autologous human peripheral blood lymphocytes. J Exp Med 1982; 155:1823-41.

31. Grohn P, Kumpulainen E, Nuortio L et al. A phase II study of metastatic melanoma treated with a combination of interferon alfa 2b dacarbazine and nimustine. Eur J Cancer 1992; 28:441-3.

32. Gutterman JU, Mavligit GM, McBride CM et al. Active imunotherapy with BCG for recurrent malignant melanoma. Lancet 1973; 1:1208-12.

33. Gutterman JU, Mavligit GM, Gottlieb J, et al. Chemoimmunotherapy of disseminated malignant melanoma with dimethyl triazeno imidazole carboxommide and bacillus calmette guerin. N Engl J Med 1974; 291:592-7.

34. Haase KD, Lange OF, Scheef W. Interferon-gamma treatment of metastasized malignant melanoma. Anticancer-Res 1987; 7:335-6.

35. Hamblin TJ, Davies B, Sadullah S et al. A phase II study of the treatment of metastatic malignant melanoma with a combination of dacarbazine, cis-platin, interleukin-2 (IL-2) and alfa-interferon (IFN). Proc ASCO 1991; 10:294(1029).

36. Hellmann K (ed). First Interleukin-2 International Symposium. Cancer Treatment Reviews. 1989; 16(Suppl A):1-176. London: Academic Press Limited .

37. Hersey P, McLeod GR, Thomson DB. Treatment of advanced malignant melanoma with recombinant interferon alfa-2a in combination with DTIC: Long-term follow-up of two phase II studies. Br J Haematol 1991; 79(Suppl 1):60-6.

38. Hersh EM, Chirigos MA, Mastrangelo MJ (eds). Augmenting Agents in Cancer Treatment. New York: Raven Press 1981.

39. Hersh EM, Gutterman JU, Mavligit GM et al. Immunocompetence, immunodeficiency, immunopotentiation and prognosis in malignant melanoma. In: Neoplasms of the Skin and Malignant Melanoma. Chicago: Yearbook Medical Publishers,1976:331-44.

40. Hersh EM, Metch BS, Muggia FM et al. Phase II studies of recombinant human tumor necrosis factor alpha (rhuTNFa) in patients with malignant disease. J Immunotherapy 1991; 10:426-31.

41. Hersh EM, Murray JL, Hong WK et al. Phase I study of cancer therapy with recombinant interleukin-2 administered by intravenous bolus injection. Biotherapy 1989; 1:215-26.

42. Hersh EM, Patt YZ, Gutterman JU et al. Host defense mechanisms in cancer and their modification by imunotherapy. In: Crispen (ed). Neoplasm Immunity: Experimental and Clinical. Elsevier/North Holland Biomedical Press, 1980:247-64.

43. Hersh EM, Quesada JR, Murphy SG et al. An evaluation of therapy with the methanol extraction residue of BCG (MER). Cancer Immunol Immunother 1982; 14:4-9.

44. Hu-Li J, Shevach EM, Mizuguchi J et al. B cell stimulatory factor 1 (interleukin 4) is a potent costimulant for normal resting T lymphocytes. J Exp Med 1987; 165:157.

45. Humphries MJ, Olden K, Yamada KM. A synthetic peptide from fibronectin inhibits experimental metastasis of murine melanoma cells. Science 1986; 233:467-70.

46. Houghton AN, Brooks H, Cote RJ et al. Detection of cell surface and intracellular antigens by human monoclonal antibodies: Hybrid cell lines derived from lymphocytes of patients with malignant melanoma. J Exp Med 1985; 158:53-65.

47. Imai K, Ng A-K, Ferrone S. Characterization of monoclonal antibodies to human melanoma-assoiated antigens. J Natl Cancer Inst 1981; 66:489-96.

48. Interleukin-2: Sunrise for immuno-therapy. Lancet (Editorial) 1989; I:308.

49. Irie RF, Matsuki T, Morton DL. Human monoclonal antibody to ganglioside GM2 for melanoma treatment. Lancet 1989; I:786-7.

50. Irie RF, Morton DL. Regression of cutaneous metastatic melanoma by intralesional injection with human monoclonal antibody to ganglioside GD2. Proc Natl Acad Sci USA 1986; 83:8694-8.

51. Ishihara M, Hashimoto K, DiGregorio FM et al. Monoclonal antimelanoma antibodies IKH-1 and IKH-2 which work on formalin-fixed, paraffin embedded tissues: Characterization, clinical trials and comparative studies with HMB-45. J Dermatol Sci 1992; 3:13-25.

52. Jotereau F, Pandolfino MC, Boudart D et al. High-fold expansion of human cytotoxic T-lyphocytes specific for autologous melanoma cells for use in immunotherapy. J Immunother 1991; 10:405-11.

53. Kahn M, Sugawara H, McGowan P et al. CD4+ T cell clones specific for the human p97 melanoma-associated antigen can eradicate pulmonary metastases from a murine tumor expressing the p97 antigen. J Immunol 1991; 146:3235-41.

54. Kan-Mitchell J, Imam A, Kempf RA et al. Human monoclonal antibodies directed against melanoma tumor-associated antigens. Cancer Res 1986; 46:2490-6.

55. Kellokumpu-Lehtinen P, Nordman E. Combined interferon and vinblastine treatment of advanced melanoma and renal cell cancer. Cancer Detection and Prevention 1988; 12:523-9.

56. Kellokumpu-Lehtinen P, Nordman E, Toivanen A. Combined interferon and vinblastine treatment of advanced melanoma: Evaluation of the treatment results and the effects of the treatment on immunological functions. Cancer Immunol Immunother 1989; 28:213-17.

57. Kim TS, Russell SJ, Collins MK, Cohen EP. Immunity to B16 melanoma in mice immunized with IL-2-secreting allogeneic mouse fibroblasts expressing melanoma-associated antigens. Int J Cancer 1992; 51:283-9.

58. Kirkwood JM. Studies of interferons in the therapy of melanoma. Semin Oncol 1991; 18(5 Suppl 7):83-90.

59. Kirkwood JM, Ernstoff MS. The role of interferons in the management of melanoma. In: Nathanson L (ed). Management of Advanced Melanoma. New York: Churchill Livingston, Inc., 1986:209.

60. Koeppler H, Pflueger KH, Seitz R, Havemann K. High-dose chemotherapy without autologous bone marrow support in advanced malignant melanoma. Onkologie 1989; 12:277-9.

61. Kradin RL, Lazarus DS, Dubinett SM et al. Tumour-infiltrating lymphocytes and interleukin-2 in treatment of advanced cancer. Lancet 1989; 3:577-80.

62. Kriazan Z, Murray JL, Hersh EM et al. Increased labeling of human melanoma cells in vitro using combinations of monoclonal antibodies recognizing separate cell surface antigenic determinants. Cancer Res 1985; 45:4904-9.

63. Larson SM, Brown JP, Wright PW. Imaging of melamona with l-131-labeled monoclonal antibodies. J Nucl Med 1983; 24:123-9.

64. Lazarus HM, Herzig RH, Graham-Pole J et al. Intensive melphalan chemotherapy and cryopreserved autologous bone marrow transplantation for the treatment of refractory cancer. J Clin Oncol 1983; 1:359-67.

65. Legha SS, Papadopoulos NE, Plager C et al. Clinical evaluation of recombinant interferon alfa-2a (Roferon-A) in metastatic melanoma using two different schedules. J Clin Oncol 1987; 5:1240-6.

66. Legha S, Plager C, Ring S et al. A phase II study of biochemotherapy using interleukin-2 (IL-2) + interferon alfa-2A (IFN) in combination with cisplatin (C) Vinblastine (V) and DTIC (D) in patients with metastatic melanoma. Proc ASCO 1992; 11:343(1179).

67. Legha S, Ring S, Plager C et al. Biochemotherapy using interleukin-2 (IL-2) + interferon alfa 2-A (IFN) in combination
with cisplatin (C) vinblastine (V) and DTIC
(D) in advanced melanoma. Proc ASCO
1991; 10:293(1024). (Abstract)

68. Leong SPL, Granberry ME, Zhou YM et
al. Selection of cytotoxic T lymphocytes
against autologous human melanoma
from lymph nodes with metastatic
melanoma using repeated in vitro
sensitization1. Clin Expl Metastasis
1991; 9:301-17.

69. Lienard D, Lejeune FJ, Ewalenko P. In
transit metastases of malignant melanoma treated by high dose rTNF alpha
in combination with interferon-gamma
and melphalan in isolation perfusion.
World J Surg 1992; 16:234-40.

70. Livingston PO, Kaelin K, Pinsky CM et
al. The serologic response of patients
with stage II melanoma to allogeneic
melanoma cell vaccines. Cancer 1985;
56:2194-200.

71. Livingston PO, Natoli EJ, Claves MJ et
al. Vaccines containing purified GM2
ganglioside elicit GM2 antibodies in
melanoma patients. Proc Natl Acad Sci
USA 1987; 84:2911-15.

72. Lotem J, Shabo Y, Sachs L Regulation of
megakaryocyte development by inter-
leukin-6. Blood 1989; 74:1545-51.

73. Mandanas R, Schultz S, Scullin D et al.
Phase II trial of cimetidine in metastatic
melanoma. A Hoosier Oncology Group
trial. Am J Clin Oncol 1991; 14:397-409.

74. Margolin K, Doroshow J, Akman S et al.
Treatment (Rx) of advanced melanoma
with cisdiammine dichloroplatinum
(CDDP) and alpha interferon (aIFN). Proc
ASCO 1990; 9:277(1074). (Abstract)

75. Margolin KA, Rayner AA, Hawkins MJ
et al. Interleukin-2 and lymphokine-
activated killer cell therapy of solid tumors:
Analysis of toxicity and management guidelines. J Clin Oncol 1989; 7:486-98.

76. Matsui M, Temponi M, Ferrone S. Characterization of a monoclonal antibody-
defined human melanoma-associated

antigen susceptible to induction by immune interferon1. J Immunol 1987;
139:2088-95.

77. Mavligit GM, Hersh EM, McBride CM.
Lymphocyte blastogenic responses to
autochthonous viable and non-viable
tumor cells. J Natl Cancer Inst 1973;
51:337-43.

78. Mazumder A, Rosenberg SA. Successful
immunotherapy of natural killer-resistant established pulmonary melanoma
metastases by the intravenous adoptive
transfer of syngeneic lymphocytes activated in vitro by interleukin 2. J Exp
Med 1984; 159:495-507.

79. McLeod GRC, Thomson DB, Hersey P.
Recombinant interferon alfa-2a in ad-
vanced malignant melanoma. A phase I-
II study in combination with DTIC. Int
J Cancer Suppl 1987; 1:31-35.

80. Merimsky O, Inbar M, Shiloni E et al.
Sequential treatment of melanoma patients who progressed on interleukin-2
and dacarbazine by a-interferon and
dacarbazine - a preliminary report. Mol
Biother 1990; 2:208-10.

81. Meyskens Jr FL, Kopecky K, Samson M
et al. A phase III trial of recombinant
human interferon-gamma (IFN) as adjuvant therapy of high risk malignant
melanoma (MM). Proc ASCO 1991;
10:291(1019). (Abstract).

82. Mickiewicz E, Estevez R, Rao F et al.
Interferon alfa 2b (rIFNa 2b) alone or in
combination with DTIC in metastatic
melanoma (MM). Compiled data. Proc
ASCO 1990; 9:281(1089). (Abstract)

83. Mier JW, Vachino G, van der Meer JW
et al. Induction of circulating tumor
necrosis factor (TNF alpha) as the mechanism for the febrile response to interleu-
kin-2 (IL-2) in cancer patients. J Clin
Immunol 1988; 8:426-36.

84. Milstein C. From antibody structure to
immunological diversification of immune
response. Science 1986; 213:1261-68.

85. Mitchell MS. Attempts to optimize active specific immunotherapy for melanoma.
Intern Rev Immunol 1991; 7:331-47.

86. Mitchell MS, Kempf RA, Harel W et al. Effectiveness and tolerability of low-dose cyclophosphamide and low-dose intravenous interleukin-2 disseminated melanoma. J Clin Oncol 1988; 6:409-24.

87. Mittelman A, Chen, ZJ, Yang H et al. Human high molecular weight melanoma-associated antigen (HMW-MAA) mimicry by mouse anti-idiotypic monoclonal antibody MK2-23: Induction of humoral anti-HMW-MAA immunity and prolongation of survival in patients with stage IV melanoma. Proc Natl Acad Sci USA 1992; 89:466-70.

88. Moertel CG, Fleming TR, Macdonald JS et al. Levamisole and fluorouracil for adjuvant therapy of resected colon carcinoma. N Engl J Med 1990; 322:352-8.

89. Morinaga Y, Hidtoshi H, Takeuchi A, Onozaki K. Antioproliferative effect of rhinterleukin1-b (rhiL-1b) on tumor cells: Go-G. Arrest of a human melanoma cell line by IL-1. Biochem Biophys Res Comm 1990; 173:186.

90. Morton DL, Bauer RL, Hunt KK, Lee JD. Immunotherapy by active immunization of the host using nonspecific agents. Section 24.1 clinical applications using intralesional therapy. In: DeVita Jr VT, Hellman S, Rosenberg SA, eds. Biologic Therapy of Cancer. Philidelphia: JB Lippincott Company, 1991:627-42.

91. Morton DL, Eilber FR, Malgrem RA et al. Immunological factors which influence response to immunotherapy in malignant melanoma. Surgery 1970; 68:158-64.

92. Mosmann TR et al. T-cell and mast cell lines respond to B-cell stimulatory factor-1. Proc Natl Acad Sci USA 1986; 83:5654.

93. Mulder NH, DeVries EG, Sleijfer DT et al. Dacarbazine (DTIC), human recombinant interferon alpha 2a (Roferon) and 5-fluorouracil for disseminated malignant melanoma. Br J Cancer 1992; 65:303-4.

94. Mulder NH, Willemse PHB, Schraffordt-Koops HS et al. Dacarbazine (DTIC) and human recombinant interferon alpha 2a (Roferon) in the treatment of disseminated malignant melanoma. Br J Cancer 1990; 62:1006-7.

95. Mule JJ, McIntonsh JK, Jablons DM, Rosenberg SA. Antitumor activity of recombinant interleukin 6 in mice. J Exp Med 1990; 171:629-36.

96. Murphy PM, Lane HC, Gallin JI et al. Marked disparity in incidence of bacterial infections in patients with the acquired immunodeficiency syndrome receiving interleukin-2 or interferon-gamma. Ann Intern Med 1988; 108:36-41.

97. Murray JL, Hersh EM, Rosenblum MG et al. Radioimmunoimaging in malignant melanoma using 111 In-labeled monoclonal antibody 96.5. Cancer Res 1985; 45:2376-81.

98. Murray DR, Cassel WA, Torbin AH et al. Viral oncolysate in the management of malignant melanoma: II clinical studies. Cancer 1977; 40:680-6.

99. Murray JL, Rosenblum MG, Lamki L et al. Clinical parameters related to optimal tumor localization of indium-111-labeled mouse antimelanoma monoclonal antibody ZME-018. J Nucl Med 1987; 28:25-33.

100. Nitta T, Oksenberg JR, Rao NA, Steinman L. Predominant expression of T cell receptor Va7 in tumor-infiltrating lymphocytes of uveal melanoma. Science 1990; 249:672-4.

101. Nowak J, Cohen EP, Graf Jr LH. Cytotoxic activity toward mouse melanoma following immunization of mice with transfected cells expressing a human melanoma-associated antigen. Cancer Immunol Immunother 1991; 33:91-6.

102. Ochoa JB, Curti B, Peitzman AB et al. Increased circulating nitrogen oxides after human tumor immunotherapy: Correlation with toxic hemodynamic changes. J Natl Cancer Inst 1992; 84:864-7.

103. Oettgen HF, Old LJ. The history of cancer immunotherapy. In DeVita Jr

VT, Hellman S, Rosenberg SA, eds. Biologic Therapy of Cancer. Philidelphia: JB Lippincott Company, 1991:87-119.

104. Onazabik, Matsushinak, Aggarwal B, Oppenheim J. Human interleukin 1 is a cytocidal factor for several tumor cell lines. J Immunol 1985; 135:3962.

105. Oratz R, Dugan M, Harris M et al. A randomized trial of an adjuvant polyvalent melanoma antigen vaccine with or without cyclophosphamide in patients with malignant melanoma. Proc ASCO 1989; 8:228(1124). (Abstract)

106. Oratz R, Speyer JL, Wernz JC et al. Antimelanoma monoclonal antibody-ricin A chain immunoconjugate (XMMME-001-RTA) plus cyclophosphamide in the treatment of metastatic malignant melanoma: Results of a phase II trial. J Biolog Response Modifiers 1990; 9:345-54.

107. Parkinson DR, Abrams JS, Wiernik PH et al. Interleukin-2 therapy in patients with metastatic malignant melanoma: A phase II study. J Clin Oncol 1990; 8:1650-6.

108. Parkinson DR, Fisher RI, Rayner AA et al. Therapy of renal cell carcinoma with interleukin-2 and lymphokine-activated killer cells: Phase II experience with a hybrid bolus and continuous infusion interleukin-2 regimen. J Clin Oncol 1990; 8:1630-6.

109. Patt YZ, Hersh EM, Schafer LA et al. The need for immune evaluation prior to thymosin containing chemoimmunotherapy for melanoma. Cancer Immunol Immunother 1979; 7:131-6.

110. Plager C, Bowen JM, Fenoglio C et al. Adjuvant immunotherapy of MD Anderson Hospital (MDAH stage III-B malignant melanoma with newcastle disease virus oncolysate). Proc ASCO 1990; 9:281(1091). (Abstract)

111. Plantefaber LC, Hynes RO Cell 1989; 56:281-90.

112. Pinsky CM, Hirshaut Y, Oettgen HF. Treatment of malignant melanoma by intratumoral injection of BCG. Natl Cancer Inst Monogr 1973; 39:225-8.

113. Porgador A, Brenner B, Vadai E et al. Immunization by gamma-IFN-treated B16-F10.9 melanoma cells protects against metastatic spread of the parental tumor. Int J Cancer (Suppl) 1991; 6:54-60.

114. Quesada JR, Talpaz M, Rios A et al. Clinical toxicity of interferon in cancer patients: A review. J Clin Oncol 1986; 4:234-43.

115. Quirt IC, Shelley WE, Pater J et al. Improved survival in pateints with poor-prognosis malignant melanoma treated with adjuvant levamisole: A phase III study by the national cancer institute of Canada clinical trials group. J Clin Oncol 1991; 9:729-35.

116. Redman BG, Flaherty L, Chou TH et al. Sequential dacarbazine/cisplatin and interleukin-2 in metastatic melanoma: Immunological effects of therapy. J Immunotherapy 1991; 10:147-51.

117. Richards JM, Gilewski TA, Ramming K et al. Effective chemotherapy for melanoma after treatment with interleukin-2. Cancer 1992; 69:427-9.

118. Richards J, Mehta N, Schroeder L, Dordal A. Sequential chemotherapy/immunotherapy for metastatic melanoma. Proc ASCO 1992; 11:346(1189). (Abstract)

119. Richner J, Cerny T, Joss RA et al. A phase II study of continuous subcutaneous alpha 2b interferon (IFN) combined with cisplatin (CDDP) in advanced malignant melanoma (MM). Proc ASCO 1990; 9:280(1085). (Abstract)

120. Rosenberg SA, Lotze MT, Muul LM et al. A progress report on the treatment of 157 patients with advanced cancer using lymphokine-activated killer cells and interleukin-2 or high-dose interelukin-2 alone. N Engl J Med 1987; 316:889-97.

121. Rosenberg SA, Lotze MT, Muul LM et al. Observations on the systemic administration of autologous lymphokine-activated killer cells and recombinant interleukin-2 to patients with metastatic cancer. N Engl J Med 1985; 313:1485.

122. Rosenberg SA, Lotze MT, Yang JC et al. Experience with the use of high-dose interleukin-2 in the treatment of 652 cancer patients. Ann Surg 1989; 210:474-85.

123. Rosenberg SA, Packard BS, Aebersold PM et al. Use of tumor-infiltrating lymphocytes and interleukin-2 in the immunotherapy of patients with metastatic melanoma. A preliminary report. N Engl J Med 1988; 319:1676.

124. Rossen RD, Crane MM, Morgan AC et al. Circulating immune complexes and tumor cell cytotoxins as prognostic indicators in malignant melanoma. A prospective study of 53 patients. Cancer Res 1983; 43:422-9.

125. Rosenstein M, Ettinghausen SE, Rosenberg SA. Extravasation of intravascular fluid mediated by the systemic administration of recombinant interleukin-2. J Immunol 1986; 137:1735-42.

126. Ruiter DJ, Matijssen V, Broecker EB, Ferrone S. MHC antigens in human melanomas. Cancer Biology 1991; 2:35-45.

127. Saleh MN, Khazaeli MB, Wheeler RH et al. Phase I trial of the chimeric anti-GD2 monoclonal antibody ch14.18 in patients with malignant melanoma. Hum Antibodies Hybridomas 1992; 3:19-24.

128. Seftor REB, Seftor EA, Gehlsen KR, et al. Role of the avb3 integrin in human melanoma cell invasion. Proc Natl Acad Sci USA 1992; 89:1557-61.

129. Severinson E, Naito T, Tokumoto H et al. Interleukin 4 (IgG1 induction factor): A multifunctional lymphokine acting also on T cells. Eur J Immunol 1987; 17:67-72.

130. Shabo Y, Lotem J, Rubinstein M et al. The myeloid blood cell differentiation-inducing protein MGI-2A is interleukin-6 Blood 1988; 72:2070-3.

131 Shiloni E, Pouillart P, Janssens J et al. Sequential dacarbazine chemotherapy followed by recombinant interleukin-2 in metastatic melanoma. a pilot multicentre phase I-II study. Eur J Cancer Clin Oncol 1989; 25:S45-S49.

132. Siegel JP, Puri RK. Interleukin-2 toxicity. J Clin Oncol 1991; 9:694-704.

133. Sosman JA, Kohler PC, Hank JA et al. Repetitive weekly cycles of interleukin-2. II. Clinical and immunologic effects of dose, schedule and addition of indomethacin. J Natl Cancer Inst 1988; 80:1451-61.

134. Spitler LE. A randomized trial of levamisole versus placebo as adjuvant therapy in malignant melanoma. J Clin Oncol 1991; 9:736-40.

135. Spitler LE, del Rio M, Khentigan A et al. Therapy of patients with malignant melanoma using a monoclonal anti-melanoma antibody-ricin A chain immunotoxin.1 Cancer Res 1987; 47:1717-23.

136. Starnes Jr HF, Hartman G, Torti F et al. Recombinant human interleukin-1b (IL-1b) has anti-tumor activity and acceptable toxicity in metastatic malignant melanoma. Proc ASCO 1991; 10:292 (1023) (Abstract)

137. Steffens TA, Bajorin DF, Houghton AN. Immunotherapy with monoclonal antibodies in metastatic melanoma. World J Surg 1992, 16:261-9.

138. Steiner A, Wolf C, Pehamberger H. Comparison of the effects of three different treatment regimens of recombinant interferons (r-IFNa, r-IFNg and r-IFNa + cimetidine) in disseminated malignant melanoma. J Cancer Res Clin Oncol 1987; 113:459-65.

139. Stoter G, Aamdal S, Rodenhuis S et al Sequential administration of recombinant human interleukin-2 and decarbazine in metastatic melanoma: A multicenter phase II study. J Clin Oncol 1991; 9:1687-91.

140. Tchekmedyian NS, Tait N, Van-Echo D, Aisner J. High-dose chemotherapy without autologous bone marrow transplantation in melanoma. J Clin Oncol 1986; 4:1811-18.

141. Tefany FJ, Barnetson RS, Halliday GM et al. Immunocytochemical analysis of the cellular infiltrate in primary

regressing and non-regressing malignant melanoma J Invest Dermatol 1991; 97:197-202.

142. Temponi M, Gold AM, Ferrone S. Binding parameters and idotypic profile of the whole immunoglobulin and Fab' fragments of murine monoclonal antibody to distinct determinants of the human high molecular weight-melanoma associated antigen. Cancer Res 1992; 52:2497-503.

143. Thatcher N. Recombinant interleukin-2 and other types of treatment of advanced malignant melanoma. Current Opinion Oncol 1991; 3:364-76.

144. Thatcher D, Lind M, Morgenstern G et al. High-dose, double alkylating agent chemotherapy with DTIC, melphalan or ifosfamide and marrow rescue for metastatic malignant melanoma. Cancer 1989; 63:1296-302.

145. Thatcher N, Wagstaff J, Mene A et al. Corynebacterium parvum followed by chemotherapy (Actinomycin D and DTIC) compared with chemotherapy alone for metastatic malignant melanoma. Eur J Cancer Clin Oncol 1986; 22:1009-14.

146. Thomson D, Adena M, McLeod GRC et al. Interferona-2a (IFN) does not improve response or survival when added to dacarbazine (DTIC) in metastatic melanoma: Results of a multi-institutional Australian randomised trial QMP8704. Proc ASCO 1992; 11:343(1177). (Abstract)

147. Vadhan-Raj S, Cordon-Cardo C, Carswell E et al. Phase I trial of a mouse monoclonal antibody against GD3 ganglioside in patients with melanoma: Induction of inflammatory responses at tumor sites. J Clin Oncol 1988; 6:1636-48.

148. Van der Bruggen P, Traversari C, Chomez P et al. A gene encoding an antigen recognized by cytolytic T lymphocytes on a human melanoma. Science 1991; 254:1643-7.

149. Van Snick J Interleukin-6: an overview. Ann Rev Immunol 1990; 8:253-78.

150. Veronesi U, Adamus J, Aubert C, et al. A randomized trial of adjuvant chemotherapy and immunotherapy in cutaneous melanoma. N Engl J Med 1982; 307:913-16.

151. Vlock DR, Kirkwood JM. Serial studies of autologous antibody reactivity to melanoma: Relationship to clinical course and circulating immune complexes. J Clin Invest 1985; 76:849.

152. Wadler S, Einzig AI, Dutcher JP et al. Phase II trial of recombinant alpha-2b-interferon and low-dose cyclophosphamide in advanced melanoma and renal cell carcinoma. Am J Clin Oncol 1988; 11:55-9.

153. Wallack MK, Steplewski Z, Koprowski H, et al. A new approach in specific, active immunotherapy. Cancer 39:560-4.

154. West WH, Tauer KW, Yannelli JR et al. Constant-infusion recombinant interleukin-2 in adoptive immunotherapy of advanced cancer. N Engl J Med 1987; 316:898-905.

155. Wolff SN, Herzig RH, Fay JW et al. High-dose thiotepa with autologous bone marrow transplantation for metastatic malignant melanoma: Results of phase I and II studies of the North American Bone Marrow Transplantation Group. J Clin Oncol 1989; 7:245-9.

156. Yang HM, Reisfeld RA. Doxorubicin conjugated with a monoclonal antibody directed to a human melanoma-associated proteoglycan suppresses the growth of established tumor xenografts in nude mice. Proc Natl Acad Sci USA 1988; 85:1189-93.

157. Zbar B, Bernstein ID, Rapp HJ. Suppression of tumor growth as the site of infection with living bacillus Calmette-Guerin. J Natl Cancer Inst 1971; 46:831-9.

INDEX